BEATING PROSTATE CANCER WITHOUT SURGERY

Beating
Prostate Cancer
WITHOUT
Surgery

James D. Priest, M.D.

With a foreword by Archbishop Desmond Tutu

Published by Fairview Press, 2450 Riverside Avenue, Minneapolis, MN 55454. Fairview Press is a division of Fairview Health Services, a community-focused health system, affiliated with the University of Minnesota, providing a complete range of services, from the prevention of illness and injury to care for the most complex medical conditions. For a free current catalog of Fairview Press titles, call toll-free 1-800-544-8207, or visit our Web site at www.fairviewpress.org.

Library of Congress Cataloging-in-Publication Data
Priest, James D.
  Beating prostate cancer without surgery / James D. Priest ; with a foreword by Desmond
Tutu.
    p. cm.
  Includes bibliographical references and index.
  ISBN-13: 978-1-57749-153-8 (alk. paper)
  ISBN-10: 1-57749-153-X (alk. paper)
  1. Priest, James D. 2. Prostate—Cancer—Patients—Biography. 3. Prostate—Cancer—
    Popular works. I. Title.
  RC280.P7P64 2005
  362.196´99463´0092--dc22

                        2005016510

Printed in the United States of America
First printing: September 2005
09 08 07 06 05   6 5 4 3 2 1

Cover by Laurie Ingram Design (www.laurieingramdesign.com)
Medical illustration by David Mottet

To my wife, Ilka—
my partner, my supporter, my lover, throughout life
and through the trials this disease made me confront

CONTENTS

Foreword by Archbishop Desmond Tutu ix

Preface xi

Acknowledgments xiii

Journal 1–149

Articles

    What Is the Prostate Gland? 7

    What Is a PSA Test? 12

    Needle Biopsy of the Prostate Gland 18

    What Is a Gleason Score? 24

    What Is Cancer? 30

    Dealing with the Diagnosis 36

    Roles of Physicians and Patients in Treating Prostate Cancer 42

    Prostate Cancer: A Bewildering Disease 48

    How Does Radiation Therapy Work? 54

Brachytherapy (Radioactive Seeds) for Prostate Cancer 60

Radical Prostatectomy: Surgical Removal of the Prostate Gland 66

Hormonal Treatment for Prostate Cancer 72

Cryotherapy (Freezing) for Prostate Cancer 78

What Is Watchful Waiting? 84

If Treatment Fails—What Next? 90

Living with Prostate Cancer 96

Erectile Dysfunction (Impotence) Following
    Prostate Cancer Treatment 102

What Do Tomatoes, Vitamin E, and Oily Fish Have
    in Common? 108

Complementary and Alternative Treatments
    for Prostate Cancer 114

Emerging Technologies for Treating Prostate Cancer 120

Afterword 151

Glossary 159

Resources 163

Index 165

Foreword

This book is a blend of emotion and education. Expressing one's self is vital, and Dr. Priest takes us on an emotional journey, telling of his shock at receiving the diagnosis of prostate cancer, the arduous process of making a decision on treatment, the treatment itself, and life thereafter.

A number of therapies exist, each with advantages and disadvantages. None is perfect or the others would not survive, and all this is overwhelming to a patient. While addressing this fact, *Beating Prostate Cancer without Surgery* also provides solid medical information on specific aspects of prostate cancer. Twenty brief articles cover subjects from the basic "What Is Cancer?" to budding research and new treatments.

As Dr. Priest points out, other than skin cancer, prostate cancer is the most prevalent cancer in American men. One of every 6 will develop it, and its highest occurrence and lowest survival rates are among African-American males.

Once diagnosed, each man must decide which treatment is best. He may research it by himself, as did Dr. Priest, but he should also seek help from health care professionals, aware that they tend to recommend procedures they themselves perform, having utmost confidence in them.

But the important thing is to be diagnosed. Visit your doctor and take the recommended tests. If found early, prostate cancer is treatable and curable, and not necessarily with dreaded complications. In most cases you have time to make decisions, so explore beyond the first opinion. If the disease is diagnosed early, you can be in control, making choices from knowledge rather than out of fear. This book can help you gain that knowledge.

And there is life after prostate cancer, I am proof of that!

Archbishop Desmond Tutu

PREFACE

This book is, first, a personal diary about my experiences, feelings, and choices after being diagnosed with prostate cancer. Second, it is an informational guide for those who have the disease or wish to learn more about it.

Whom is this book meant for? The 1 out of 6 men who will develop prostate cancer, of course. But also their partners, and here's why.

When a physician tells a man he has prostate cancer, the man is often stunned, overwhelmed, and confused, and may comprehend little of what's said next. He may lapse into a period of shock or denial lasting days or even weeks during which he is unable to think clearly or make rational judgments.

But important decisions have to be made, and it's often the partner and other loved ones in the man's life who gather the information and help him make an appropriate decision about what to do.

All prostate cancer treatments can lead to complications, the major ones being incontinence (inability to hold urine) and impotence (inability to perform sexually). Incontinence is a serious problem, but it can be dealt with. For many men, impotence (also known as erectile dysfunction) is a more complicated and intractable problem. Impotence—sometimes temporary, sometimes permanent—is historically a common complication of prostate cancer treatment. If a couple is prepared for this possibility ahead of time, they may be able to deal with it more easily, both individually and as a couple. Additionally and more importantly, it is helpful to know in advance that some treatments are better than others at preserving sexual function.

The information in this book will be useful for anyone coping with prostate cancer. Whether you yourself have just been diagnosed with the disease, or you want to better understand and support someone else who has prostate cancer, this book is for you.

Acknowledgments

For helping me cope with my disease, I am greatly indebted to my family: my wife, Ilka; sons, David and Eric; brother Jack; and cousin Ellen.

For their assistance, I am grateful to Archbishop Desmond Tutu and his personal assistant, Lavinia Browne; radiation oncologist Tae Kim, M.D.; and my friend Bob Bodsgard. Thanks, too, to the physicians and staff who treated my cancer and continue to follow my progress.

Special thanks to Jeffrey K. Cohen, M.D., Director, Division of Urology, Allegheny General Hospital, Pittsburgh, and Associate Professor, Surgery, Drexel University College of Medicine, Philadelphia, Pennsylvania, who reviewed and contributed to the article on cryotherapy; to John D. Wilson, Ph.D., Associate Professor of Radiology, Medical College of Virginia, for his help on how radiation affects cells; and to Khalil Ahmed, Ph.D., University of Minnesota, for his assistance with the article on emerging technologies.

And thanks to Lane Stiles, Director of Fairview Press, who skillfully edited this book.

Except for myself and members of my family, the names of the people in this journal have been changed to protect their privacy.

BEATING PROSTATE CANCER WITHOUT SURGERY

Monday October 23

"You have cancer in your prostate," says Dr. Fitzgerald.

Four months earlier I'd had a physical exam before knee surgery. "We've got to do the routine screening tests," said my family doctor, an old friend. "It's just common sense. At your age you need a colonoscopy to rule out bowel cancer and a PSA, a blood test, to rule out prostate cancer."

My wife, Ilka, had been after me for years to have these tests done. But I knew I didn't have cancer. I was too healthy, too happy, too busy. And here's a cliché: I never thought it would happen to me.

I went ahead with the PSA, and the result was 4.5. The upper limit of normal is 4.0. My family doctor referred me to a urologist, Dr. Fitzgerald.

"The PSA is a prostate-specific test," he said, "not a prostate cancer-specific test. It can go up from sexual activity, prostatitis, riding a bike, and a few other things."

"Then it doesn't mean I have cancer," I said, relieved.

"Not at all. To clear up any prostatitis—inflammation or infection of the prostate gland—I'll put you on an antibiotic, and we'll get another PSA and see whether it's come down."

I took the antibiotic for three weeks and didn't get around to having a second PSA drawn for several more weeks. Was I afraid of what the result might be? I was busy. I didn't have cancer anyway, I told myself.

Dr. Fitzgerald phoned. "The second PSA is 4.9. You can go on another course of antibiotics or have a biopsy of your prostate."

The physician in me took charge. "I'll have the biopsy," I said.

The biopsy was done in his office using a rectal probe that projects needles, one after another, into the prostate gland. For me, it was uncomfortable but not really painful. Eight needles went in, each withdrawing a section of gland. Those sections were examined under a microscope, which revealed cancerous cells.

When Dr. Fitzgerald calls and says, "You have cancer in your prostate," I am stunned. I put my wife on the phone with me.

"Prostate cancers are given a Gleason score," he says. "Yours is 6. The higher the score, the more aggressive the tumor. Yours is moderate in severity. But it's cancer."

Except for skin cancers, prostate cancer is the most common cancer in American men. In 2005, over 232,000 new cases will be diagnosed in the United States.

He discusses the forms of treatment, mainly surgery and radiation. "I do not recommend radiation," he says. "I recommend surgery, radical prostatectomy. It's the gold standard for treating prostate cancer. The main complications are incontinence and impotence. You're in the hospital for three or four days and must wear a catheter in your bladder for a few weeks."

"When can you do it?" asks my wife.

"I'll be out of town for a while," he says.

"When will you be back?" I ask. I have cancer. I want it out of my body.

"In a couple of weeks," he says. "But other doctors in this office do the operation."

We get off the phone, bewildered and upset. I'm 62 years old, I think. Will this shorten my life? Am I going to die? "Incontinence" means the inability to hold your urine. "Impotence" means the inability to perform sexually. It doesn't sound good at all.

Ilka comes to me and hugs me. "We'll get through this like we have everything else."

Anxiously I go onto the Internet, search for information on prostate cancer, print out articles, and together we read them.

Thus begins our investigation into the diverse world of prostate cancer.

Tuesday October 24

I don't want to write this journal. I'm a novelist, and right now one of my characters is stranded in an underground cavern. I guess she'll have to stay there until I can get back to her. Right now I have something else to attend to.

So why am I writing the journal? Writing is a way I make sense of life, and I'm hoping that writing will somehow help me deal with this.

I phone my older brother, Bob, in Arizona and tell him. "I'm so sorry to hear that," he says. "But I'll tell you one thing. Whatever treatment you choose, look around and find a doctor you have confidence in and get along with, because you'll be seeing an awful lot of him."

My younger brother, Jack, a retired pediatric oncologist, is out of town. I try to get hold of him and leave a message.

I phone Steve, whose prostate cancer was operated on by Dr. Fitzgerald three years ago.

"I'm doing well," he says, "but I still wear a pad when I play tennis because I drip with exercise or activity. If you want the names of several other men who've had prostate cancer, I'll give them to you. Three live right on our block."

Three on his block? I take the names.

I phone my family physician, who has referred me to Dr. Fitzgerald. "I have prostate cancer," I say.

"I know," he says. "The urologist called me yesterday before he called you."

"Why did he call you?"

"He knew you and I go way back, and he felt terrible about the cancer. I'm really sorry you have to go through this. But at your age and with the tumor found early, you should probably have surgery."

"Maybe so. I'm starting to research the condition."

My wife and I are assured from our reading that the cure rate and longevity are good if this cancer is caught early, which mine has been. Treatment has improved markedly. They say most men nowadays don't die of prostate cancer, they die with it.

It's a more common cancer than we thought. One out of six men in the United States has it. That's astounding. No wonder many think that the PSA test should be universally administered.

How do I feel? Frightened, depressed, dreading the surgery—should I decide to have surgery. According to the information we're reading, surgery can cause incontinence for weeks, months, or even years, and, more frighteningly, results in impotence at least half the time.

Ilka and I walk around the lake. She takes my hand. We discuss the doctors' appointments I have scheduled and the bone scan Dr. Fitzgerald has recommended. It is a dark, gloomy day, exactly matching my frame of mind.

Wednesday October 25

A spider lives on and around my computer. I've been regularly undoing its attempts to build webs on my desk. The spider is on my computer this morning when I turn it on and skitters away when the screen lights up. Do spiders have prostates? Get cancer? I hope not. I wouldn't wish cancer on any other living thing.

I hope to see Dr. Fitzgerald in the next couple of days to discuss treatment in more detail. I'm preparing a list of questions for him: What types of surgery are available? How many operations has he performed? What are the potential complications of prostate surgery? What is the average rate of these complications overall? What is the rate for the surgeries that Dr. Fitzgerald has performed himself? What is the risk of infection from the catheter? How effective are supplements such as selenium and vitamin E? (My cousin heard a report that they can be helpful.) Will the cancer spread through my body if I bend over or move around?

Cancer. I cringe to think/say/type the word. Cells in my body are growing out of control and are going to cause me a whole lot of trouble.

We had plans to go to Florida in three weeks. The plans are scuttled.

Still, I try to look on the bright side of things. Recently I was on a diet. Yesterday, due to my stress over the diagnosis, I ate nothing until dinner. I might lose a little weight. Hmm. My middle feels a little smaller already.

> In a lifetime, 1 man in 6 will develop prostate cancer, while 1 woman in 7 will have breast cancer.

Three months ago I had a complication from knee surgery. The joint filled with blood the day after the operation and had to be drained. It's taken me a long time to recover. The knee was just starting to feel good when this new problem arose.

And knee surgery is something I understand. As an orthopedist, I did knee surgeries for many years. But I know nothing about prostate surgery, except that it's a big abdominal operation with the potential for many complications. I don't even want to think about it.

But I must.

How do I feel today? Somewhat depressed but calmer. Thank God for Ilka and my friends. I wouldn't want to face this alone.

I play tennis with three male friends. One knows I have prostate cancer, and I tell the other two. I play pretty well, but am depressed, distracted.

One reason my family doctor has referred me to a urologist is that I have urinary urgency. When I have to go, I have to go. That's just the way it is.

"Well," I joke with the other players, "incontinent and wearing a diaper, I won't have to worry about urgency any more." They don't think the joke is funny.

I come home and spend the rest of the day researching prostate cancer on the Internet.

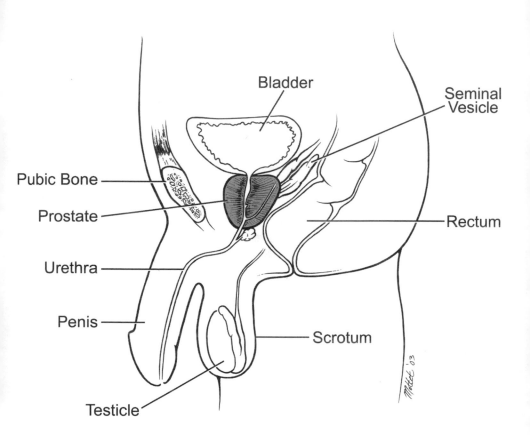

Bladder

Seminal
Vesicle

Pubic Bone

Prostate

Urethra

Penis

Testicle

Rectum

Scrotum

What Is the Prostate?

The size of a pea in a baby boy, the prostate begins growing at puberty until it is walnut- or plum-sized. The often troublesome gland resides behind the pubic bone, above the base of the penis, below the bladder, and in front of the rectum. Running through it is the upper portion of the urethra, the tube which carries urine from the bladder to the outside world.

A gland is an organ secreting fluid for use elsewhere in the body or for elimination from the body. In the female, the breast gland produces milk. In the male, the prostate secretes a milky white fluid that nourishes sperm cells and is discharged with them in the ejaculate.

The ejaculate—or semen—is made up of sperm from the testes and fluid produced partly in the prostate. The prostate gland consists of thousands of microscopic channels, and sacks bulging off of them, which are lined by cells producing the fluid. Surrounding them is a muscular wall that contracts during ejaculation and helps propel the semen on its way down the urethra.

Cells lining the prostate's ducts and bulges also produce large amounts of PSA, whose purpose is to liquefy the medium about the sperm cells enabling them to swim freely. Some PSA leaks through the walls of blood vessels traversing the prostate and can be detected in a PSA blood test.

According to prostate pathologist Dr. Jonathan Oppenheimer, the breast and prostate, both hormonally influenced glands, are made up of cells and channels appearing remarkably similar under a microscope. It is interesting to note that, with the exception of skin cancer, breast cancer is the most common cancer in American women, and prostate cancer is the most common cancer among American men.

Thursday October 26

Ilka drives me to the hospital so that I can be injected with radioactive dye for a bone scan. She waits as I register and sign a release document. Then another patient and I make our way to Nuclear Medicine together, just before noon. In the waiting room we hand the receptionist our paperwork. She looks at his, then at her schedule.

"Your appointment's at 2:00 o'clock," she says.

"Oh, I was told noon," he says. Puzzled, he turns and leaves.

"Is mine at noon?" I ask.

"Yes," she says, "and it's already been called back."

"Does that mean I should go back there?" I ask, pointing toward the area behind her where injections are given.

"Oh, no," she says summarily.

I sit down, unsure.

She leaves, and another receptionist takes over. Ten minutes later the new one glances at me, then at my paperwork.

"Are you Dr. Priest?" she asks. I nod.

She picks up the phone. Whatever is supposed to have been "called back" hasn't been. But a technician soon comes out and calls my name. I stand up. "Come with me," she smiles.

She escorts me into Nuclear Medicine's inner sanctum and sits me down in a small room.

I ordered many a bone scan for patients while I was practicing orthopedics, but I never thought I'd need one myself. Being on the other side of the desk—being the patient—is not something I am relishing.

"What are you going to inject me with?" I ask.

"Technetium," she says, preparing my hand for the injection, "a radioactive isotope."

"How long will it be in my body?"

"Theoretically, forever. It has a half-life of 6 hours—half is gone in 6 hours, another half in 6 more, and so on."

"So that next little half will always be there, inside me, getting smaller and smaller."

"That's right. The isotope passes out in your urine."

I have visions of my toilet bowl aglow in the middle of the night. "Will I be putting anyone else at risk with this radioactivity in my body?"

"No, we don't even consider it a risk to you."

She deftly inserts a needle through the skin on the back of my hand. I watch as a clear fluid is injected into me. Removing the needle, she covers the puncture with a small bandage.

A hospital wristband with the name of a physician I do not recognize is on my wrist. "Who's the doctor whose name is on my wristband?"

A radioactive isotope, or radioisotope, is a compound that gives off radiation as its atoms decay, or break up. This radiation is easy to detect with certain kinds of medical equipment and so allows medical specialists to see things inside the body that they would not otherwise be able to see.

She looks quizzically at it, then at the same name on my papers. "I don't know of a physician by that name—or whether he even exists. We'll have to get the right doctor, or your report might be sent to someone else."

Three errors have been made in the first few minutes of my expedition into caring for my cancer. This doesn't fill me with confidence.

A patient—any patient, even a doctor who's a patient—needs to be alert at all times. If there's an obvious error, like the one on my wristband, it must be pointed out right away.

Ilka and I return home to wait for the radioactive dye to circulate through my body. As we arrive, a man in a spacesuit is spraying trees in our next door neighbors' yard. The chemicals, I think, must be hazardous for him to be wearing the kind of outfit he is wearing. What if the material comes over onto our property? Could it give us cancer?

Then I remember. I already have cancer. It's still hard for me to say this, think this.

I look up at a dark sky. As if the sun knows, I think. It hasn't been out since I learned my diagnosis.

While waiting at home for the radioactive dye to circulate, I continue my research on prostate cancer.

What's a bone scan? When prostate cancer spreads, it frequently goes to bone, often the pelvis and lower spine. Technetium is a radioisotope that, during a scan, reveals hot spots in the bones where the cancer has spread. Dr. Fitzgerald has ordered the test not because he fears my cancer had spread, but because he wants a baseline for future reference.

My son David, a physician in California, tells me by phone that a family friend has just been treated for prostate cancer. I'll try contacting him.

"Do you know how common prostate cancer is?" asks David. "The risk increases with age. I heard in medical school that 80 percent of 80-year-olds have it, and 100 percent of men living to be 100 have it."

"That's pretty common," I say.

> Exceeded only by lung cancer, prostate cancer is the second leading cause of cancer death in men in the United States, where almost 30,000 men will die of it in 2005. Prostate cancer accounts for about 10 percent of cancer-related deaths in men.

Back to the hospital at 3:00 for the bone scan. I've been instructed to drink lots of fluids between the injection and the scan, and I have dutifully consumed four or five tall glasses of water and urinated three times, all the while worrying about the drive back to the hospital. (I haven't forgotten my urinary urgency.)

We make it back to the hospital with no unfortunate accidents. But my concern about my bladder is a precursor of many episodes to come.

A plump technician enters the waiting room. "Dr. Priest?" she says. I stand up. She glances at my wife. "He'll be back in 15 minutes."

Escorting me back to the scanning chamber, she asks, "Do you have keys, coins, or metal of any kind on you?"

"No," I say, wondering why she asks.

In the scanning room she asks again.

"No," I repeat, putting my hands into my pockets. "Why?"

"It would distort the scan," she says.

I certainly don't want that.

She helps me lie down on a table on my back. "I'm claustrophobic," I say.

Her response is hardly reassuring. "The machine will start right in front of your face and move slowly down toward your feet. You must lie as still as possible." She walks to the other side of the room and starts the machinery.

Staring point blank at the machine, trying to remain calm and motionless, I hear a song in my head. I share a quirk with my son Eric. A tune comes to mind and repeats itself over and over, whether we like it or not. My dad taught me the one I hear now.

> Oh, there was an old man named Michael Finnegan,
> Who had some whiskers on his chinnegan,
> The wind came out and blew them in-again,
> Poor old Michael Finnegan. Begin again!
> There was an old man named ...

As the song goes on, I realize that "Finnegan" has changed to "Mil-i-ken." Michael Milken, the famous junk bond dealer, developed prostate cancer and used, among other things, diet to treat it. He has a large web site dedicated to the disease. It is obvious what is on my mind.

After the machine passes by my head I can see the ceiling, and I wonder why they don't put a picture or poem or something for the patient to gaze at while trying to lie completely still.

Just about the time I conclude the scan is over, the technician leaves the room. I don't know whether I am allowed to move or if I must continue lying still. I am disturbed by this uncertainty, but a few minutes later she reappears. She gets me up, takes me to a waiting room, and says they will now check the films for quality.

What Is a PSA Test?

It is important to detect prostate cancer early. The earlier the cancer is detected, the more treatable it is.

The two most common assessments for early detection are the digital rectal exam and the PSA blood test. The PSA blood test is especially important for detecting prostate cancer. A cancer can grow in the prostate for years before it can be detected by a digital rectal exam. A PSA test can detect cancer much sooner.

PSA stands for "prostate-specific antigen." Prostate-specific antigen is an enzyme secreted by the microscopic channels and clusters of cells in the prostate gland. Prostate tissue is the only tissue in the body that can produce it.

PSA is normally in high concentration in the semen and in low concentration in the blood. But it can leak into the blood, and thereby become detectable with the PSA test, when something happens to the prostate. That something can be prostate cancer, but frequently it is something else: pressure, inflammation, or some other factor that compromises the gland's structure or integrity. The PSA test, then, is a prostate-specific blood test, not a prostate cancer-specific test.

Factors that can elevate the level of PSA in the blood include:
- Inflammation or infection of the prostate (prostatitis)
- Prostate swelling (benign prostatic hyperplasia, or BPH)
- Urinary tract infection
- Ejaculation within the last 48 hours
- Bicycle riding
- Needle biopsy of the prostate

It is not clear whether a digital rectal exam elevates the level of PSA in the blood, but as a precaution it is recommended that blood be

drawn for a PSA test before such an exam rather than after.
The PSA test measures the number of nanograms of prostate-specific antigen per milliliter of blood. A value of up to 4.0 nanograms per milliliter (ng / ml) is considered normal.

Who should have a PSA test? The American Cancer Society advises health care professionals to offer a digital rectal exam and PSA yearly beginning at age 50 to men who have a life expectancy of 10 years or more. For men in two high-risk categories—African Americans and men with a first-degree relative (father, brother, son) diagnosed with prostate cancer at an early age—testing should begin at age 45.

Men at even higher risk (i.e., those having several first-degree relatives diagnosed with prostate cancer at an early age) could begin testing at age 40. Depending on this initial test's result, further testing might not be required until age 45.

The American Cancer Society advises health care professionals to provide their patients opportunities to openly discuss the benefits and risks of testing and encourages men to actively participate in the discussion by learning about prostate cancer and its early detection and treatment.

Not everyone agrees that routine testing is desirable, and many scientific and medical organizations do not support routine PSA testing for prostate cancer. Scientists at the National Cancer Institute (NCI) are studying whether certain cancer screening tests actually reduce cancer deaths. Though the trial is ongoing, preliminary results suggest that men who have a very low PSA value might not need to be retested every year.

In a study in the May 28, 2003, *Journal of the American Medical Association*, researchers at Memorial Sloan-Kettering Cancer Center found that the PSA commonly fluctuates above and below "normal" levels. Of nearly a thousand men who had 5 consecutive PSA tests in a 4-year period, 21 percent had a PSA level above 4.0 ng / ml at some point during the study. But when these same men were retested a year or more later, nearly half had normal PSA values, which, in most cases, remained normal during further testing.

The PSA test can produce both false positive results and false negative results. A "false positive" PSA test means the level of PSA in the blood is elevated, yet cancer is not present. A "false negative" test means that the PSA value is normal even though cancer is present. Therefore, the PSA test should be repeated at regular intervals.

According to the American Academy of Family Physicians, of 100 men who have a PSA test, 10 will have a value above normal. For 3 of these 10 the elevated PSA will be caused by prostate cancer. For the other 7 the cause will be something else. Of the 90 men with a normal PSA, one will have prostate cancer.

What should the level of PSA in the blood be after treatment for prostate cancer? If the gland is surgically removed, the PSA test should be zero, because no prostatic tissue should remain in the body. After radiation through implanted radioactive seeds or external beam, the PSA should be low and remain stable, as it should after any form of treatment. After cryotherapy, the accepted value for success is 0.4.

After any treatment for prostate cancer, a PSA test should be done annually for at least 15 years.

I look down at my sandals. They have metal clasps on them. Nervously I envision having to reshoot all the film.

She returns, smiling. "The films are fine."

It has been much longer than 15 minutes by the time I get back to the waiting room. On the way to the car, Ilka and I meet some longtime friends. The woman is being treated for cancer. The coincidence is a reflection of the stage in life we have all reached.

In the evening I phone my son and several friends. "I'm in my study. All the lights are out, and radiation man's aglow. I could read a book in here." Gallows humor.

We'll see the urologist tomorrow morning for a discussion of treatment options. He'll recommend radical prostatectomy. He already has, when he called with the diagnosis. My family physician has advised surgery also. But I'll have a surgeon's worst nightmare in my hand tomorrow: a list of questions about surgery from another surgeon.

We'll also find out whether this cancer has spread to bone.

Friday October 27

We are escorted into Dr. Fitzgerald's office. A tall man with sandy hair, he comes through the door shaking his head. "I don't have the bone scan results. It hasn't even been read, but I've got a call in to a radiologist."

He sits down behind his desk. As we wait we chat. "Some other things might show up on the scan," I say. "I've had surgery on both knees, most recently the left, and pain in my right foot."

The phone rings and Dr. Fitzgerald answers it. It is the hospital radiologist. Dr. Fitzgerald listens quietly. I look away, afraid of reading something into his facial expression. He hangs up. "You have early arthritis in your joints. Your left knee surgery shows up, and so does the problem in your right foot. Prostate cancer can spread to the lumbar spine and pelvis. There's no sign of that."

I am greatly relieved. The tumor hasn't spread to bone. Hopefully, it is confined to the prostate.

We talk at length about treatment options, the two major ones being surgery and radiation, and the possible complications of treatment.

"Your Gleason Score is 6," he says. "But one of the reasons I'm recommending prostatectomy is that it's not uncommon for the Gleason Score to go up once we've removed the prostate and can look at the whole gland under a microscope. In other words, your tumor might be more aggressive than we can tell from the needle biopsies. Another reason I recommend surgery is that after radiation surgery's not really an option. The radiated area is scarred and difficult to operate on. But—if needed—radiation is an option after surgery."

A recent study suggests that "salvage" surgery—in this case, surgery after radiation therapy has failed to kill the prostate cancer—may be an option after all.

I ask about surgical alternatives, including laparoscopic prostatectomy, and the staging, or progression, of my disease. I ask about the possibility of infection from the catheter I would have to wear postoperatively; about selenium, vitamin E, and alternative therapies; about "watchful waiting," the preferred course of action in older men.

"Could it spread," I ask, "by my bending over, or being active, such as playing tennis?"

"No," he says.

"Can cancer cells in my urine transmit the disease to someone else?"

"No."

I ask about surgeons and surgeries, about how many prostatectomies he has done, and about his cure and complication rates. He is thorough in his discussion, which includes the possible complications of incontinence and impotence.

"We have ways of treating impotence," he says. "Viagra, vacuum devices, injections, implants. You can have sex with your prostate gone. But men tell me it feels different—pleasurable, but different."

Different? I think.

"What if the cancer's been treated with surgery and radiation," I ask, "and comes back?"

"We put you on hormones," he says, "and that suppresses it for five years."

Then what? I wonder. It sounds as if that's it. After that you're on your own.

Ilka mentions our friend Steve. "You did a prostatectomy on him three years ago."

"Ah, yes," he says. "I consider him one of my successes."

He dribbles when he plays tennis, I recall. Did he wet the bed after his catheter came out? Is he able to function sexually?

"What assurances are there," I ask finally, "that the biopsy slides with my name on them are indeed mine, that those prostate specimens came from me?"

He has answered all my other questions to the best of his ability, but this one stumps him. I don't think anyone's asked him this before.

Mistakes are made in medicine, several yesterday before my scan. Once when I was still practicing medicine, I walked into an operating room where a doctor I knew was doing surgery. He looked up at me. "I'm operating on the wrong hip," he said. He was halfway through the operation before the mistake was discovered.

Now I'm a patient, and I don't want mistakes made on me.

Dr. Fitzgerald's nurse calls into his office by intercom. "Should I phone the hospital and say you'll be late for surgery?"

He says yes. We've been with him for almost an hour. I have a few more questions, and he takes his time answering them.

When we leave I feel better, though not unreservedly so. After all, I have newly diagnosed cancer and I'm not certain what to do about it.

We go to the mall to shop for clothes for the upcoming weekend. I think I am hungry, but when we sit down for lunch my appetite isn't there. I become very tired, and after 3-1/2 hours am glad when we start for home.

Poor me. Why me? As a child I had polio, so why cancer, too?

Needle Biopsy of the Prostate Gland

If detected early, prostate cancer is usually a highly treatable disease. Typically, early detection of prostate cancer involves routine screening using digital rectal exams and PSA blood tests. If the prostate gland feels enlarged, irregular, or nodular when examined rectally, or if the PSA is elevated and other noncancerous conditions that can cause it to be elevated have been excluded, a prostate biopsy might be in order.

Biopsy of the prostate is a common procedure performed by a urologist in his or her office. With the patient lying on an examining table, the urologist inserts a lubricated ultrasound probe into the patient's rectum. Using the ultrasound image of the prostate for direction, the urologist places multiple small spring-loaded needles one by one through the thin rectal wall into the gland. Each needle is in the prostate for only a fraction of a second, but retrieves a slender core of prostatic tissue.

The whole procedure takes about 15 minutes and can be done without an anesthetic. If necessary, a local anesthetic gel can be used to reduce discomfort. In my case the procedure was uncomfortable but not overly painful. Prior to the procedure an enema clears the bowel.

The number of needles used, and therefore the number of sections taken, is usually between 6 and 12. The specimens are sent to a pathologist, who evaluates them under a microscope.

Infection and excessive bleeding are possible complications of the procedure, but are rare, occurring in less than 1 percent of patients. The patient should consult with his physician about any blood-thinning medications he may be taking, such as aspirin and anti-inflammatories. He should also let his physician know if he is taking any supplements, as these may also affect the ability of the blood to clot. The doctor will tell the patient if he should stop taking any medications or supplements before the biopsy to reduce the risk of bleeding. An antibiotic taken before and after the procedure can guard against infection.

After the biopsy, small amounts of blood may appear in the urine, feces, or semen, and may continue to be present from a few days to a few weeks.

Needle biopsy is widely used for obtaining sample sections of a prostate gland. But the operative word is "sample." Needles cannot penetrate every last recess of the gland, so it is possible to miss a cancerous area. If a patient has a negative biopsy but an elevated PSA, another biopsy might be indicated.

Saturday October 28

Ilka and I drive an hour and a half to a lodge in Wisconsin for an outing we have previously planned. On the way we talk little about my condition.

I'll see a radiation oncologist next week who implants radioactive seeds in the prostate. My brother Jack is a retired pediatric oncologist. For years he worked with a radiation oncologist whom he recommends highly. I'll try to see this specialist as well.

Sunday October 29

We drive home. I type an e-mail to two of my oldest friends. We went to college together and have remained in touch ever since. I write that I have prostate cancer, but I don't sent the e-mail. I don't want to tell them yet.

Today part of me feels, why not just do it, get it over with, whatever the course of treatment, and get back to doing the things I want to do—the things I love doing?

But part of me worries that if I rush and don't make the right decision, I may no longer be able to do things I want to do.

Monday October 30

I still have trouble saying that I have prostate cancer. This morning I'm getting back to revising my first novel. I usually enjoy doing this, but I'm a bit depressed today thinking about what lies ahead. Things aren't the same, and won't be until I get all this behind me—seeing doctors, being treated, dealing with the consequences.

I'll play tennis this afternoon because I need exercise and diversion.

I'm not as consumed with researching prostate cancer as I was at first, partly because of the cautionary example of Andy Grove, the co-founder and chairman of Intel. When Grove developed prostate cancer, he exhaustively researched the subject and chose to undergo a type of radioactive seeding, which he wrote about in a lengthy article in *Fortune* magazine. But I've since heard by word of mouth that Grove's therapy failed. Rather than trying to do everything myself, I'm going to listen to my physicians.

This evening we pick up our son Eric at the airport. He's a law student in Chicago, here for an interview with a law firm. It is the first time I've seen him since I was diagnosed. He's keenly interested and anxious.

"How are you feeling, Dad?" he asks as I pull away from the curb.

"I range from panic to depression," I say. "No, just kidding. I think I'm okay."

Tuesday October 31

We visit radiation oncologist Dr. Scott Francis.

Ilka and I are in the examining room when his nurse comes in. The first thing she says is, "This will be your only visit here. You may phone Dr. Francis, but he's not always able to respond."

This doesn't sound promising.

She interviews me for a long while, then leaves when the doctor arrives. Working with various urologists, he has done almost 1,000 prostate seedings. "The procedure is always performed," he explains, "by a radiation oncologist and a urologist together."

We go over everything, and the doctor is very forthcoming. Perhaps too forthcoming. His answer to a question from my wife shocks both of us. "If you were diagnosed with prostate cancer, what treatment would you choose?" she asks him

"I wouldn't pick external beam radiation," he answers. "The seeds work well, but if push came to shove I might choose radical prostatectomy."

Hmm. Not a very strong endorsement for the procedure he performs.

All this does is muddy the waters further. We leave in even more of a quandary about what to do than when we arrived

Before a seeding procedure, he recommends that the patient take Lupron for three months, a hormone that shuts down the male hormone testosterone. I might just opt to take Lupron and go underground for a few months to consider the options. This is not an easy deal. We take our son back to the airport.

Wednesday November 1

Nervous and upset, and on a dreary, rainy day, I go to play indoor tennis with three male friends. They are all concerned about my condition and what I am going to do. One suggests I call another tennis player who attends a monthly prostate support group.

Ilka and I go to the hospital and see a second radiation oncologist, Dr. Bruce, who has worked with my brother for 20 years and for whom Jack has the utmost respect. As seems customary with radiation oncologists, his nurse meets with us first and describes the seeding procedure.

Then Dr. Bruce comes in. He is medium height, in his fifties, slightly balding. We discuss seeds and external beam radiation, and he is thorough, gentle, knowledgeable, and likable.

"Your tumor," he says, "has been caught early. Whichever treatment you choose—external beam radiation, seeding, or radical prostatectomy—you'll do well."

I like the sound of this.

"At this hospital," he says, "we have the BAT machine and 3D conformal external beam radiation. The BAT ultrasound machine allows us to locate the

Of all prostate cancers, 86 percent are found in local and regional stages, "local" meaning still confined to the prostate gland, "regional" indicating spread to nearby areas but not distant sites in the body. The five-year relative survival rate for all these men is nearly 100 percent.

prostate gland right now, today. It can move up to a centimeter and a half from day to day depending on what's in the bladder and bowel. Without the BAT system, radiation oncologists don't know the prostate's exact position and must radiate a generous margin around it to make sure it's within the radiation beam. But in doing so they also radiate significant portions of the rectum and bladder and can cause complications like rectal bleeding and urethral narrowing.

"The 3D conformal system targets the area to be radiated better than any previous equipment. Using the two systems together, we can reduce the margin and decrease complications, yet still hit the prostate. This is the latest and best equipment. Right now no other hospital in this state has the BAT machine, but I'm sure they'll get it. I'm confident we deliver radiation as well as anyone in the country."

Ilka asks the same question she asked Dr. Francis. "What treatment would you select if you were in Jim's shoes?"

He smiles. "I can't do that because I'm not in his shoes—having to make a decision in the face of fear, worry, and a deluge of information."

She presses him for an answer.

"For your husband," he says, "I would choose seeds because that method has a longer track record than 3D conformal external beam radiation. For myself, because I'm familiar with how it works, I would choose external beam."

"Why not surgery?" she asks.

"If you've seen one man with incontinence for the rest of his life," he says, "you've seen enough."

He promises to fax me a paper on health outcomes following prostatectomy and radiotherapy, and after we get home he does. A long and complex study. I read through it with interest.

What Is a Gleason Score?

Named after its inventor, Donald F. Gleason, M.D., Ph.D., a pathologist at the University of Minnesota, the Gleason score is the most extensively used tool in the United States for rating how aggressive a case of prostate cancer may be.

The only way to diagnose cancer is by examining cells under a microscope. If a rectal exam indicates that the prostate is abnormal, or if a PSA test indicates that the levels of PSA in the blood are above normal, a biopsy of the prostate is often the next step.

The biopsy is performed through the rectum by a urologist. Several slim needles are inserted into the prostate, each removing a slender tissue core. These samples of prostate tissue are sent to a pathology laboratory where a pathologist carefully examines them under a microscope. If cancer is discovered, the pathologist determines the tumor's Gleason score based on the cancer cells' arrangement and appearance.

The score is the sum of two numbers representing the two most common cancer cell patterns. The first number represents the major or dominant pattern, and the second number the minor or secondary pattern. If 95 percent of the tumor has the same pattern, the number representing that pattern is used twice.

Both numbers range from 1 to 5, 1 signifying the most normal appearing cancer cells, 5 denoting the most aggressively malignant ones. The two numbers are added together to give the Gleason score. For example, if the dominant pattern is scored a 2 and the secondary pattern is scored a 3, the Gleason score would be 5. The Gleason score can thus range from 2 to 10. In general, the higher the score, the more aggressive the cancer.

The first of the two numbers is more important, as it represents the dominant cancer cell pattern. Thus, a 3 + 4 = 7 tumor would generally have a better prognosis than a 4 + 3 = 7 tumor, even though both have the same Gleason score.

A tumor tends to behave as its score would suggest. Those with low-end scores (2 to 4) tend to be slow-growing and not likely to spread. Those with mid-range scores (5 to 7) can be unpredictable in growth and malignant potential. Those with high-end scores (8 to 10) are the most aggressive, and the patient might have distant spread when the cancer is discovered.

Occasionally tumors behave in a fashion not corresponding with their appearance under a microscope. Some seeming low-grade might expand aggressively; others that appear fast-growing could behave benignly.

Another way to establish a Gleason score is by examining the entire prostate. A score obtained in this fashion is more accurate because all areas of the gland can be scrutinized. The score might be higher than one from slender samples, because the needles might fail to discover a more malignant cancer focus.

A Gleason score determined by examining the whole gland is one of the best predictors of the tumor's behavior. But it requires removing the prostate from the body, a procedure not every patient elects.

Thursday November 2

I telephone the tennis player from the prostate support group. "You're in the nick of time," he says. "It meets tonight. In it are men with varying problems having gone through different treatments."

Ilka and I decide to go.

"I feel better about my situation today," I tell her, "more at peace than at anytime since I learned the diagnosis. I'll decide what treatment to have and be confident about it. I'm relieved that I can talk with Dr. Bruce who seems to care about me as a patient."

Unsolicited, today Dr. Bruce faxes me another study showing that patients with a PSA of 0 to 10 have almost identical cancer-free results at eight to nine years whether they have prostatectomy, seeds, or external beam radiation.

At 7:00 o'clock we go to the support group. The meeting has been moved to an adjacent building, and by the time we find the room we are late. About 25 men and a few women are there.

The topic is incontinence. A urologist presenter shows slides of a device that can be surgically implanted if incontinence persists after prostatectomy. Encircling the urethra, it can be pumped up to stop urine leakage. Doesn't look too appealing to me.

Another speaker, a nurse who deals with incontinence, shows numerous slides of pads and devices developed to treat incontinence. Makes us think it must be quite an issue.

"Urologists vary widely in their estimates of how many post-surgery patients will be wet," she tells the audience. "The figures range from 1 percent to 30 percent."

My wife and I go up to her after her presentation. "In your experience," I ask, "what percentage of postoperative patients are incontinent?"

She thinks for a moment. "Closer to the 30-percent figure than the other."

The meeting is over, and Ilka chats with a gentleman who has had surgery and now suffers from leakage. "I'm not happy about it," he says. "If I had it to do over again, I'd probably choose seeds."

"I wear diapers," says another. "I'm thinking about having that thing put in that you pump up to stop the leaking."

A man is there with his wife. When diagnosed he'd had a PSA of 9, a Gleason Score of 8, and tumor extension beyond the prostate. "I went on Lupron," he says, "for five or six months. I had hot flashes and breast enlargement. Then I had the seeds put in, and had burning on urination for a couple of weeks until I stopped drinking caffeine and fruit juice. I just now started external beam radiation."

"Those attending these meetings," I tell Ilka as we leave, "are the ones with problems. Those doing well have no reason to come. But incontinence after surgery seems no small problem."

How many patients, I wonder on the way home, even go to another doctor after being told by a physician they have cancer? How many get a second opinion, or third? Do health plans pay for this?

Friday November 3

I'm trying to focus less on my cancer and more on my normal life, but the topic is hard to avoid. I play doubles today, and the three other men are all aware of my situation.

"Anything new?" one asks privately. "Decided what to do?"

"Not yet," I say. "I'm still thinking about it."

We join the others.

"Can you guys play on Thanksgiving morning?" asks another. He looks at me.

Telling them what I am going through isn't easy. "I have prostate cancer," I say. "I don't know if I can play, because I might be having treatment then."

"I know four other guys with prostate cancer," he says. "Seems almost normal at our age."

Saturday November 4

I speak with my family physician, an old friend.

"If your brother has worked with this radiation oncologist for 20 years," he says, "he should take really good care of you."

Sunday November 5

Walking the dogs this morning, I bump into a neighbor.

"When are you leaving town?" he asks.

"We had planned to go to Florida on November 15," I say, "but we put that on hold."

He looks at me curiously.

Over and over, I am finding that I resist telling people what I have. "I have prostate cancer, and we'll be staying here until it's treated."

Monday November 6

Only clear liquids for me today in preparation for a colonoscopy tomorrow, a test advised by my family doctor when he also recommended the PSA. I sincerely hope the results of the colonoscopy are better that those of the PSA.

It's been two weeks since I learned I have prostate cancer. I've come to accept that I've reached the time of life when medical visits will become more common.

A controversy is stirred up again today. Dr. Bruce mentioned the name of the urologist he feels comfortable working with for seed implantation. I phone to make an appointment, but the urologist's schedule is full for weeks.

I call Dr. Bruce. "Is there any chance you could help me get in sooner?"

"Instead of that," he says, "I'll call Dr. Fitzgerald, your original urologist, and ask whether he would do the procedure with me. I haven't worked with him before."

"How many seedings have you done?" I ask.

"Not nearly as many as Dr. Francis. Fewer than 100."

After talking with Dr. Fitzgerald, Dr. Bruce calls me back. "He was a bit hesitant about it and said he'll call you directly."

This troubles me.

"The other day," I say, "you told me I'd 'do well' with any of the three treatments—surgery, external beam radiation, or seeds. What did you mean by 'do well'?"

"You'd have very good chance of cure," he says.

Now I'm less troubled.

I hang up, uncertain whether Dr. Fitzgerald is hesitant about working with Dr. Bruce or about the possibility of my choosing seeds over prostatectomy. After all, Dr. Fitzgerald has recommended prostatectomy. He's probably hesitant about both.

"I'm not looking forward to him calling me and trying to persuade me to have surgery, which is what he'll doubtless do," I tell Ilka.

"Just listen politely," she says.

I read an article aloud to her, titled "New Weapons Against Prostate Cancer." Therapies that manipulate genes or suppress the supply of blood to tumors have already being done experimentally.

My brother Jack has been out of town but returns this evening. I think he'll be a big help in sorting things out. Hopefully, I'll feel comfortable making my decision soon.

Dr. Fitzgerald doesn't call. Maybe he will tomorrow.

Tuesday November 7

I'm getting ready for my colonoscopy. Have just taken my second dose of physic.

The colonoscopy's over now. It wasn't entirely comfortable, but it's done. A polyp was found, removed, and sent for analysis.

Dr. Fitzgerald doesn't call.

What Is Cancer?

The adult human body is made up of 60 trillion cells, each an integral part of the whole. But they are hardly permanent.

Except for nerve cells in the adult brain, all cells in the body divide to form two new cells. They do so to replace old cells and repair damage. Every second about a million cells in our bodies are replaced. In a year, that's about equal to the total number of cells in the human body. Without an orderly process for getting rid of cells, in a year we would double in size. Many cells, therefore, die a programmed death.

Some cells divide more frequently than others, but all—except cancer cells—do so in a disciplined and systematic fashion.

The process of division is controlled by the cell's blueprint, DNA, which instructs the cell what to do and how to do it. If the DNA of a single cell becomes deranged, or if the machinery that uses DNA to duplicate cells makes a mistake, the cell divides abnormally, its descendants divide abnormally—and cancer may result. Cancer cells divide numerous times, and each time they do they can become more abnormal.

The body has a protective mechanism, called the immune system, for searching out and destroying such deviant cells. But if the system fails, the cells can reproduce and flourish unabated.

At first the abnormal cells expand where the cancer began, and because they are so small they might reproduce for years undetected before a mass—or tumor—is discovered. But some can also enter the blood stream or pathways called lymphatics, and travel to other parts of the body, such as lymph nodes, the liver, bones, and the brain. This process is called metastasis. In their new locations, cancer cells form new malignant masses that invade and replace normal tissue, causing malfunction, pain, distress, and sometimes death.

The diagnosis of cancer can only be made by examining these minute cells under a microscope. A pathologist (a physician highly trained in this disease) scrutinizes the cells' features—their size, shape, growth patterns, and the density of stain used to prepare the tissue specimen. Normal cells are neat, clean, and uniform, growing and dividing in organized patterns. Cancer cells are bizarre, ugly, blotchy, malignant, and multiply in highly unorganized patterns.

The pathologist also evaluates the degree of malignancy. If the cells are only slightly abnormal, the disease may be mild and the prognosis for the patient may be more hopeful. If the cells are wild, misshapen, and jumbled, the disease is severe and the prognosis for the patient may be less hopeful.

Not all tumors are cancerous. Some are benign, made up of tissue not having the elements of cancer. Benign tumors do not spread to other parts of the body and are harmful only when they apply pressure to adjacent structures. A benign tumor in the skull, for example, can cause the brain to malfunction.

What causes cancer? What damages the DNA or the cell division process? There is no simple answer, but important factors are genetics and environment. Some people are born with genes predisposing them to cancer. Environmental factors, such as exposing lungs to smoke or skin to sun, are known to produce cancer.

What's incredible is that trillions of cells follow the biological rules every day. But, in the great scheme of things, what's tragically ironic is that something so tiny—a single illogical, unruly, and suicidal cell—can instigate problems so immense that in the end its host, the cell itself, and all its descendants are destroyed because it was different.

Wednesday November 8

Dark and cold outside, and I'm a bit depressed. Is it gray everywhere, or just here? My brother and I have a lengthy phone conversation, discussing seeds, external beam radiation, and surgery. We also talk about watchful waiting, which means you do nothing but keep an eye on things. It's the avenue of choice for many older men.

Frank Sanders calls to invite us for Thanksgiving dinner. I turn him down because we're going to my brother's house. "How nice to have two invitations," I tell Frank.

"Prostate cancer's in my family," he says.

"Isn't it in everyone's?"

"I've taken some stuff for years to prevent me from getting it—selenium, calcium, potash, phosphorous, manganese, and magnesium in the form of a mineral supplement. And my PSA has stayed down."

"Whatever works."

> If a close relative has prostate cancer, a man's risk for the disease more than doubles. With two relatives, the risk increases fivefold. With three close relatives, the risk is about 97 percent.

Thursday November 9

Gray and cold outside. I feel nervous and depressed, the weather closing in on us. The pain might be dulled a little if I had something to look forward to, like a warm vacation. But we're not going anywhere. We have business to attend to.

I don't know what I should do. I'm in shock—not a good feeling, but better than the terror I felt when I first learned I have cancer.

I'm considering watchful waiting and taking the sort of supplements that Frank does. Not too much calcium, though, because it can cause kidney stones. Our son Eric developed one, which led to serious problems—spiking fevers, kidney and blood infections, and a two-week hospitalization, during which he nearly died.

Eric still sees a urologist for the condition. "I mentioned your cancer to him," Eric tells me on the phone. "He said if it happened to him, he'd have the seeds. He's a urologist and wouldn't choose prostatectomy."

I give three studies about prostate cancer to my brother Jack for his review: the two Dr. Bruce faxed to me and one from *Popular Science* we picked up at the support group meeting.

Friday November 10

A friend faxes a *Consumer Reports* newsletter, a publication of Consumers Union, with a four-page summary of tests and care for prostate cancer. Regarding seed therapy, it says a study from Seattle found that men with less aggressive tumors had a recurrence rate of 40 percent after 10 years, roughly double the rate for surgery or external beam. It concludes that surgery is probably the best way to prevent recurrence. Could this summary have been put together by urologists?

It's really hard determining what treatment is best. I'm waiting for my brother to talk with Dr. Bruce.

Jack has gone over the papers I gave him. "One set of results really stuck out," he says. "In an early trial of conformal radiation with less than 100 men, an extremely high percentage were disease-free after several years. As an oncologist, that really impressed me. Those are extraordinarily favorable results for an early investigation of any new therapy."

Saturday November 11

"Anything new?" a friend asks.

"I'm closer to deciding," I say. "If I had to choose today, it would be external beam radiation."

I read about the side effects of radiation in a booklet from Dr. Bruce's office. Generally, radiation causes fatigue and skin irritation. The side effects of prostate-specific radiation include bladder and bowel irritation. But compared with the side effects of surgery, this is a picnic.

Monday November 13

Normally I don't like going to the dentist, but today is a change of pace. It's almost a relief to spend an hour and a half in the chair while health professionals work on my beleaguered torso's opposite end.

My brother calls. "I talked with Dr. Bruce by phone, and I'll visit him on Wednesday when we'll have plenty of time to talk."

I have a long phone conversation with Ilka's sister Miki about the disease and various treatment options.

Tuesday November 14

It seems strange, just sitting on this cancer, not jumping all over it. But everyone seems to think I can take my time deciding.

I delve further into the Internet, particularly looking for research about the newest form of external radiation—3D conformal external beam radiation (3D-CRT)—and about complications from the various types of treatment.

Complication rates are high with radical prostatectomy—9 to 30 percent of patients experience incontinence, and 60 to 80 percent experience impotence.

There are fewer significant complications with permanent seed implants than surgery, but the potential complications can still be consequential. Radiation-induced impotence can develop over time, occurring in about 25 percent of all patients. Rates of incontinence are very low, affecting about 1 percent of patients. Other urinary symptoms, such as pain or difficulty urinating, increased frequency, and decreased urinary stream, occur in around 30 percent of patients, but newer techniques may reduce the rates of such complications. These urinary symptoms tend to dissipate over time, but can last as long as a year or two. Four to 5 percent of patients may require surgical intervention for urinary obstruction. Rectal complications, such as burning, pain, and diarrhea, occur in less than 5 percent of patients.

And, though it doesn't seem to happen often, seeds can migrate.

After researching for three weeks, I'm leaning toward conformal external beam radiation for the following reasons:

(1) In one study, 91 percent of 188 men were disease-free 3 to 8 years after treatment.

(2) In a study of 357 men given high-dose radiation, 97 percent did not experience a spread of the cancer to other parts of the body, 99 percent did not die from prostate cancer, and 96 percent were relapse-free after three years.

(3) In a good-prognosis, high-radiation group, most recurrences occurred within the first three years.

(4) A recent Mayo Clinic study found that cancer recurred in nearly 30 percent of the men who'd had radical prostatectomies.

(5) Dr. Bruce said that because my disease is early I have a very good chance of being cured no matter which of the three major treatments—surgery, seeds, or external beam radiation—I choose.

(6) If Dr. Bruce had prostate cancer, he would elect external beam radiation for himself.

(7) External beam radiation is the least invasive of the three major treatments, and I fear complications from the others, including infection.

(8) External beam radiation has fewer long-term urinary complications than surgery or seeds.

(9) "Cold spots" (areas that radiation treatment misses) can occur with seed therapy.

Dealing with the Diagnosis

The first few days after learning I had cancer were awful. I was shocked, frightened, numbed. A series of questions raced through my mind in an obsessive loop. Am I going to die? If so, how do I make the most of what time I have left? How do I make sure that my family's needs are taken care of after I'm gone?

My urologist, who did the biopsy and informed me of the cancer, recommended surgery. So did my family physician, a trusted friend and associate. At first I was all for it. I had cancer, cells in my body multiplying and expanding out of control. I wanted the cancer out.

But bad things can happen during surgery. I'm a surgeon. I know. The average man knows there are risks. His surgeon tells him that. But the average man doesn't know everything that can happen and, believe me, doesn't want to. Three months earlier I'd had "routine" knee surgery and developed a serious complication. Hospitals harbor bacteria that can cause serious, even untreatable, infections.

According to the national Centers for Disease Control and Prevention, hospital infections are the 4th leading cause of death in the United States, after heart disease, cancer, and stroke. The Chicago *Tribune* reports that these infections kill more people each year than car accidents, fires, and drowning combined.

Even if the surgery went well, I would be wearing a catheter in my bladder for weeks and might be incontinent for weeks or months— possibly for the rest of my life.

I'd wear a diaper wherever I went, whatever I did. Would I have to carry extra pads in my briefcase, in my car's glove compartment? Where and how would I dispose of the soaked ones? Would there be an odor? Could the pads leak? Would I have to curtail my social and physical activities ?

And what about impotence, another major complication of prostate cancer surgery? How would I feel knowing that I couldn't get an erection ever again without using a pump, an injection, or a pill? These thoughts were alarming and depressing.

Imagine the humiliation and insecurity that incontinence and impotence can cause, threatening both the public and private aspects of a man's life—perhaps permanently.

When I first learned I had cancer, my thoughts were irrational and peculiar—not a good time to be making life-shaping decisions. I was worried about wearing a diaper, but at the same time I told my cousin, "I don't care about impotence. I just want the cancer out."

I'm not sure when it happened, but at some point I shifted from being a passive patient—listening to everybody, believing everybody—to an active decision-maker. Many patients with cancer, unfortunately, don't make this transition.

As a doctor, I know that surgery is often the most effective way—sometimes the only way—to treat certain conditions. Appendicitis, for example, requires surgery. And a patient should generally approach surgery with confidence and resolve. After all, most patients do not acquire an infection in the hospital.

But I also know that there is often more than one way to treat a problem. My research into prostate cancer, for example, taught me that if the cancer is found early enough, there are nonsurgical options as effective as surgery but with fewer risks.

My cancer was diagnosed early. I had time to consider the alternatives. I did. And when I finally decided on treatment, I was relieved. "The worst is over," I told my wife. "What?" she asked. "Making the decision," I said.

But I'm claustrophobic and worry about how confining it might be under that radiation machinery.

Ken, a good friend, phones from Arizona. He's 80 years old. "I can only think of one friend who's not had prostate cancer," he says, "and they've all done well no matter what treatment they selected."

This is encouraging.

Wednesday November 15

My brother meets with Dr. Bruce, oncologist to oncologist. Afterwards I talk with Dr. Bruce briefly on the phone. We'll meet tomorrow.

Thursday November 16

I go back to Dr. Bruce, who examines me, including doing a digital rectal exam.

"I find no nodules in your prostate," he says, "and your disease is early."

"I am leaning toward 3D-CRT," I say.

He simply nods.

"What are the long-term complications?" I ask.

"Because the rectum and bladder are very near the prostate," he says, "external beam radiation to the prostate can cause long-term problems in those other organs. One to 5 percent of patients develop incontinence, some of it stress incontinence—patients lose a little urine picking up a heavy object or jumping on the tennis court. A urethral stricture will occur in 1 or 2 percent of cases. One to 5 percent develop slight rectal bleeding—blood on the toilet tissue after a hard stool—

The urethra is the tube that carries urine from the bladder. In men it also carries semen. A stricture is a narrowing of a tube that restricts flow. Therefore, a urethral stricture is a narrowing of the urethra that restricts the flow of urine.

which can be helped by a stool-softening diet. But once that condition develops, there's no cure for it. The patient will probably have to live with it the rest of his life, though it's extremely rare to be life-threatening. But these urinary and rectal complication rates are all from employing older radiation techniques, not 3D-CRT."

I show him some of the literature I've been studying.

One article is from a 1998 study at the University of Michigan. Patients suitable for radical prostatectomy—that is, with early stage, localized prostate cancer were treated with 3D-CRT with these results:

- The survival rate at both 5 and 8 years was 95 percent.

- Five deaths occurred, none from prostate cancer.

- 85 percent of the patients experienced no rise in their PSA levels after 8 years.

- Eight years after treatment, the results were at least as good as surgery.

- The stability of the results between 5 and 8 years was encouraging. There were no deaths between 5 and 8 years.

- The study concluded that 3D-CRT was an excellent option for patients with early prostate cancer.

Researchers at the Mayo Clinic in Rochester, Minnesota, found that cancer recurred in nearly 30 percent of 2,700 men who'd had radical prostatectomies for prostate cancer that had not spread from the prostate to other parts of the body. The study's results were given in the August 2000 issue of the journal *Urology*. Horst Zincke, M.D., a Mayo Clinic urologist, wrote, "We found the highest rate of recurrence during the first three years after radical prostatectomy." He added, "A significant number of men also had disease progression ... five years after surgery."

The following somber statement about radical prostatectomy is on the website of the American Foundation for Urologic Disease: "About 1 of every 200 to 400 men die from complications, such as heart attacks or blood clots, that are related to the operation."

Death? I thought incontinence and impotence were bad.

A 1999 study from the Fox Chase Cancer Center in Philadelphia found no difference in rectal urgency and urinary incontinence between men treated for prostate cancer with 3D-CRT and healthy age-matched men from the general population.

"What about impotence?" I ask. We hadn't discussed it.

"The impotency rate after 3D-CRT is still under investigation," he says. "With older radiation equipment it was around 50 percent. Another study from the Fox Chase Cancer Center seems to indicate that with 3D-CRT it's not that high."

I had read a summary of this study as well. The six-year study demonstrated excellent post-3D-CRT sexual function in men with prostate cancer who were 65 years old or younger. Three years after treatment, 73 percent were potent compared to 85 percent potency in men of the same age in the general population. Six years after treatment, 59 percent were potent compared to 78 percent potency in men of the same age in the general populace.

That's it for long-term complications from external beam radiation. Not so bad. There appear to be fewer complications than from seeds or surgery—and apparently with similar outcomes.

A recent study suggests that external beam radiation for prostate cancer may increase the risk of developing rectal cancer. Data for this study, however, were collected before such new technologies as IMRT came into use. Please consult your physician about this matter.

I leave Dr. Bruce's office and go to my brother's house. We talk at length about his visit with Dr. Bruce yesterday and mine today, as well as my literature search. I am embarrassed discussing impotence with his 19-year-old daughter in the background. She brings her dad a cup of tea. I decline.

Friday November 17

After almost four weeks I make a decision. I call Radiation Oncology and speak with a therapist. "I'd like to go ahead with external beam radiation."

"We'll schedule you for a planning session," she says.

I'm not sure what that means.

I phone my brother and tell him what I've decided. "Do you have any objections or second thoughts?" I ask.

"None," he says. "It seems a proper choice."

We have luncheon guests: my older brother's wife, Sherry, and daughter, Marti. The conversation around the dining room table is, not surprisingly, about you-know-what.

"My stepfather," says Marti, "had radiation for throat cancer, as did a breast cancer patient I know."

"Did they have fatigue during the radiation?" I ask. "That's one thing that can happen."

"Both did."

"How bad was it?"

"The kind of thing where they carried on their daily lives, but rested more than usual. You know, it's a time to let others do things for you."

I guess I'm in for that. But with long-term complication rates so low, I'll just deal with it.

Roles of Physicians and Patients
in Treating Prostate Cancer

There is often more than one way to treat a medical problem, and this is certainly true for prostate cancer. Different kinds of doctors will recommend different kinds of treatments.

When a routine blood test revealed that the PSA in my blood was elevated, my family physician referred me to a urologist, a doctor who specializes in the urinary organs in males and females and the sexual organs in males, for further examination.

After a second blood test confirmed that my PSA was above normal, the urologist recommended a biopsy to check for prostate cancer. A few days after the biopsy, I was stunned to learn that I had cancer.

Urologists are surgeons. It's how they're trained, it's how they make their living; and most urologists quite naturally believe that surgery is the best way to treat prostate cancer. My urologist recommended surgery for me.

But other specialists also treat cancer, and they may or may not recommend surgery. A medical oncologist, for example, treats cancer with hormonal therapy, biological therapy (or immunotherapy), and chemotherapy. A radiation oncologist treats cancer with radiation.

What do various specialists typically advise for treating prostate cancer? Researchers from Harvard, the University of Massachusetts, and the University of Connecticut asked more than 1000 doctors what they would recommend for a typical prostate cancer patient. Is it surprising that their study, as reported in *Harvard Men's Health Watch* in March, 2002, found that 93 percent of the urologists recommended surgery and 72 percent of the radiation oncologists recommended radiation?

How can you, as a patient, decide what treatment is best for you if your physician, however well-intentioned, is biased toward one particular type of treatment?

The most important thing you can do is to obtain more than one medical opinion—and from more than one medical specialty. Be sure to ask each specialist the risks, side effects, and complications of any treatment you are considering.

Second, you need to gather the most current information you can about prostate cancer. This book is a start, but you should also take a look at some of the other resources listed at the back of this book and do additional research on your own.

Third, talk with other men with prostate cancer. What did they choose to do and why? What were their outcomes? How satisfied are they with the choices they made? If they had it to do all over again, would they make the same decision? Why or why not?

Remember that no method of treatment is perfect. No method can boast 100 percent success rates. No method can guarantee there won't be complications or side effects. At some point you, the patient, must take the bull by the horns, make your best judgment, and commit fully to a choice of treatment.

Saturday November 18

On the way to play tennis I have a chilling experience. We have an older car with rear-wheel drive. Not good for winter driving when roads are slippery, as they are today. I come up over a curving freeway bridge and—going 55 miles an hour and with traffic all around—the rear wheels spin out and I have no control of the car. I'm certain that I am going to crash or roll over and the other vehicles are going to hit me. Inexplicably, though, the car straightens out and I go on, happy to be alive. A small miracle, and I am sure glad of it. I think to myself, will I have a similar happy ending with the prostate cancer treatment I've chosen? Will radiation therapy straighten me out and keep me alive?

After tennis I tell the guys that if they need an extra player this winter to fill their games I'll be around.

I watch football feeling relieved that at least I've made a decision.

We live by a lake, and today our arm of the lake is frozen over. Dr. Bruce says the radiation will take 8-1/2 weeks. I'm here for the duration.

We have a pre-Thanksgiving Thanksgiving celebration for our older son David, who has come home for the weekend from California. We're having a pre-Thanksgiving celebration because he has to work on the real Thanksgiving Day. Our friends Carol, Phil, Susan, and Rich and Ilka's sister Miki are here. Ilka makes a sumptuous dinner of turkey, stuffing, salad, wild rice, cranberry sauce, mashed potatoes, and two deserts—pecan pie without the pecans and chocolate cake. I haven't been eating much the past month since learning of you-know-what. But I take two helpings of this feast.

People are unusually sympathetic around me nowadays. I'm not sure how to react to that.

Sunday November 19

On my computer I've been putting articles and information about prostate cancer into a folder called "Ca." This morning I clean up the computer desktop. Among other things, I move the "Ca" folder to my hard drive so it will no longer be staring me in the face.

Winter's closing in on me. Light outdoors is getting shorter (so is life). The thermometer outside my window says 26 degrees. In two to three weeks I'll be starting treatment: 8-1/2 weeks of radiation, which won't be finished until mid-February. These little tumor cells are going to produce a long winter for me.

But I check the five-day weather forecast on AOL and—lo and behold—some sunshine and a warming trend are predicted over the next few days.

A lot of tension when you're in a decision-making, life-affecting struggle like I am.

Our faithful old dog almost bites me when I try to displace him so that I can lie down on the couch. This is going to be one hell of a bad three-month period—period.

Tuesday November 21

I'm up at 4:19 in the morning looking at a beautiful crescent moon. We may have some sun today.

11:40 a.m. We do have sun, a rarity this month. I'm feeling more comfortable having made a decision about treatment, and hope I can move on to other things in life.

I speak with Dr. Bruce by phone. "If the tumor has spread," I ask, "will the radiation take care of that?"

"I think you have a localized condition that hasn't spread," he says. "But if the tumor has migrated to the lymph nodes, the radiation wouldn't treat that."

"I understand that approaches like gene therapy and tumor blood vessel inhibition are experimental now, but perhaps won't be in the future. After radiation can other forms of therapy like these be used?"

"Yes, that's not a problem."

Thursday November 23

Thanksgiving Day. A lovely day weather-wise (blue skies) and family-wise.

Among American men diagnosed with prostate cancer, racial or ethnic variations are striking. The occurrence among black men (180.6 per 100,000) is more than 7 times that among Koreans (24.2). Indeed, blacks in the United States have the highest rates of this cancer in the world. African-American men have about a 60 percent higher incidence of prostate cancer than white men, and about a two-fold higher mortality rate than white men. Asian and native American men have the lowest incidence rates.

At 1:00 we go to my brother Jack's house for dinner with family and friends. Each holiday in his home, before eating we stand hand in hand around the sagging, food-laden table, and sing, "Oh, the Lord is good to us!"

A close relative has been recently diagnosed with lung cancer that has spread to the liver, a very serious illness. He's in the VA Hospital.

Today, before the song, my brother makes an announcement. "You all know Nouli's father has cancer." Jack glances at me. "Jim has a mild form of cancer, too."

Friday November 24

Bright, sunny morning. This time of year when the sun is out, it's low in the southern sky. When I sit at the computer, I face south-looking windows. In the morning I wear a baseball cap to keep the sun's rays from beaming unimpeded into my eyes. But—to have sun—I'll gladly tolerate this.

Now that I've settled on a course of treatment, I realize what a lucky stiff I am—and for lots of reasons. I came into this healthy and strong. I have a supportive wife and family. My kids are grown, educated, and doing well. I have many good friends. We live in a nice house in a friendly neighborhood. We're comfortable enough financially that I can focus entirely on my condition.

Being a doctor, and having a brother who's a doctor—in fact, an oncologist—I've had a lot of advantages in learning about this disease compared to most men who get it. I worry about these men, many of whom are getting one-sided information from their physicians and, for one reason or another, are not seeking a second opinion. Perhaps they are ignorant of their options. Maybe they are afraid or embarrassed. Maybe they lack money or health insurance. Perhaps they are already in poor health or lack supportive relationships.

If it is this hard for me, what must it be like for them?

I phone Sherry, my older brother's wife, in Kansas. Her nephew is training to become a radiation oncologist.

"He told me you made exactly the right decision in choosing external beam radiation," she says and gives me his phone number.

Prostate Cancer: A Bewildering Disease

Trying to sort through the medical information on prostate cancer can be confusing, even downright misleading, especially for a lay person. Let me give you some examples.

In a recent high-profile case, Andy Grove, the co-founder and chairman of Intel, chose a type of brachytherapy to treat his prostate cancer and wrote a widely read article about it in *Fortune* magazine. A highly respected man who did a lot of research before choosing his treatment, Grove may well have influenced other men to pursue similar treatment. What these men may not have known, however, was that Grove's therapy apparently failed and he had to turn to another form of treatment.

At a support group I attended with my wife, a urologist showed slides of a device that could be surgically implanted after prostatectomy if incontinence became a persistent problem. The device encircled the urethra in such a way as to squeeze it when the device was pumped up, thereby stopping leakage. As a surgeon, I considered implanting such a device to be a serious operation fraught with difficulties and pitfalls. But to a lay person suffering from chronic incontinence, it might have sounded like a good idea. One member of the support group said he was leaning toward having it implanted.

"Urologists vary widely in their estimates of how many post-prostatectomy patients will be wet," said another speaker at the same meeting. "The figures range from 1 to 30 percent."

From 1 to 30 percent? I thought.

"In your experience," I asked, "how many are incontinent?"

The speaker thought it over. "Closer to 30 percent," she said.

Some literature reports incontinence rates of 50 percent one year after surgery. There's a big difference between 1 chance in 2 and 1 chance in 100!

These discrepancies may reflect differences in who is doing the surgery and where the surgery is being done. But how is the average man supposed to analyze and comprehend such information? He's just been told he has cancer. Who has the knowledge, the nerve, the presence of mind to question the experience and skill of the authority figure who has just given him this news?

A recent *Consumer Reports* newsletter concludes that surgery is the best way to prevent the recurrence of prostate cancer, while an article on prostate cancer in the *New Yorker* finds no clear-cut advantage to surgery. A Michigan radiation oncologist writes that a major long-term complication of external beam radiation, occurring in about half of patients, is impotence, but a Fox Chase Cancer Center study shows excellent post-radiation sexual function in men with prostate cancer who were 65 years old or younger. One of the possible reasons for the disparity in this latter case is that the Fox Chase Cancer Center used more recent radiation equipment to treat the patients in its study. But how would an average person know this?

Here's the bottom line: Medical information can seem complex and contradictory. If you have prostate cancer, seek out more than one medical opinion. Be sure to discuss with each specialist the risks, side effects, and complications of any treatment you are considering.

Saturday November 25

Another bright morning. Baseball cap in place. The prostate thing fades somewhat into the background when you have other stuff to do and you've made your decision.

Try calling Sherry's nephew and get his answering machine.

Monday November 27

Ilka and I go to the planning session for radiation. Not knowing what to expect, I am quite nervous. First we see Dr. Bruce, then I go with a nice radiation therapist named Sally to a simulation room filled with complicated machinery. They help me lie down on a table on my back and proceed to fabricate a mold for my legs and feet.

"We'll use this every time you have treatment to keep you positioned the same each time," says Sally.

A large machine begins rotating around me taking X-rays, and the table begins to rotate as well.

Later, Sally shows me the films, and I, the nimble-witted orthopedist, note that my hip joints are normal.

Then Sally makes x's, called "crosshatches," on my skin using a permanent marker. She makes the marks above my pubic bone in front and at the same level on both hips and my back and, for protection, covers them with tape.

"This tape won't come off," says Sally, "even in the shower. We'll use the marks to position you on the treatment table with laser beams projected from various locations in the room."

Next she takes me down the hall to a CT scanning room. I am glad she is staying with me. Placing me on another table, she carefully and exactly positions me.

"We're going to take more pictures," she says. "I'll make sure they're okay and come back." She leaves the room.

As I lie perfectly still, more X-rays are taken. The procedure takes five minutes.

Sally opens the door. "The films are perfect."

I slide off the table, and she escorts me to a room in Radiation Oncology where she and a nurse sit me down and advise me on various aspects of prostate radiation. "It can irritate the rectum and bladder," says the nurse. "You can expect to have to empty them more immediately than usual."

That's a nice way of putting it, I think.

"After the treatments have been completed you might have blood in your stool for a while," says Sally. "This can also happen during therapy if there are existing problems such as hemorrhoids."

"Most patients develop radiation fatigue," says the nurse.

"Dr. Bruce will begin planning your treatment," says Sally, "and we'll call you with your first appointment."

The session is over. This is all there is to it. I'm relieved.

On the way home we stop for lunch at a Vietnamese restaurant "I think the worst is over," I tell Ilka. "Making the decision. Even with help from my brother and Dr. Bruce, and having a medical background as I searched the Internet, the decision was extremely difficult."

Fatigue seems to be the worst side effect of radiation. I'm not looking forward to it. But I most certainly wouldn't look forward to surgery, or even seeds. I'm more confident every day that I've made the right choice.

Using the X-rays taken of me today, Dr. Bruce will construct a 3D simulation of my body on the computer over the next 5 to 10 days. Then he'll use the simulation to fire trial beams to determine the best paths and angles for delivering the maximum amount of radiation to the prostate and the minimum amount of radiation to the rectum, bladder, and surrounding tissue, including bone.

The daily dose of radiation I will receive is calculated three times to be sure it's accurate—triple redundancy, just like NASA. First the amount is calculated by a dosimetrist (a radiation specialist), next by a physicist, and finally by a physician.

I receive a letter in the mail with the results of my colonoscopy. No cancer. The biopsied polyp is benign. Good news. I won't need another colonoscopy for 10 years.

Sunlight breaks through the overcast this afternoon, and we observe a pink sunset with yellowish clouds in a baby blue sky. It's about time.

Tuesday November 28

It's gray out, but for some reason I feel good.

Have just gotten back from the dentist: two fillings and a crown. The dental work is done, the colonoscopy is done. I wait to hear from Dr. Bruce's office about starting radiation.

Friday December 1

Some sun this morning, but clouding over. Still waiting to hear from Dr. Bruce.

I have a long phone conversation with Dr. Rob Tanner, Sherry's nephew, the radiation oncology fellow.

"The side effects and long-term complications of 3D-CRT are fewer than with seeds or surgery," he says, "yet the long-term results are at least as good. The operative words here are 'at least.' Those patients having only their prostates radiated just fly through treatment. Some don't even know the machine was turned on. You're making the right choice."

This is good to hear.

"I think it will become the norm for treating prostate cancer," I say.

"I believe you're right."

Tuesday December 5

"Your first treatment will be a week from tomorrow," says a therapist calling from the hospital.

I have a question for Dr. Bruce, and he comes on the line. "May I take glucosamine tablets for my joints during treatment?"

"No problem," he says. "How are you doing?"

"I'm at peace with choosing this treatment. The gold standard for prostate cancer is radical prostatectomy. But I feel external beam radiation will someday be the norm. It isn't now because it lacks longevity, hasn't stood the test of time."

"I would agree."

Friday December 8

I start radiation next week and I'm still okay with the decision.

My wife goes to a coffee get-together. The hostess's husband has undergone prostate surgery and now wears a diaper. The hostess doesn't think it's a big deal, but her husband is quite embarrassed about it.

Saturday December 9

My cancer treatment begins on Wednesday, and I have one thing and one thing only on my mind: scorching those malignant prostate cells. Alarming to think that malicious cells can lurk in your body.

"Why aren't the healthy organs radiated when the prostate is?" asks Ilka.

"They are, of course," I say, "but presumably and hopefully the precise targeting of the 3D-CRT and BAT systems steers that radiation away from good tissues and concentrates it on the bad. Dr. Bruce is working hard—maybe even at this moment—to make that happen. We simply have to trust."

How Does Radiation Therapy Work?

What does radiation therapy do? How does it kill cancer cells, and what effect, if any, does it have on other cells in the body?

The human body is comprised of trillions of cells. Except for nerve cells in the brain in adults, all cells in the body go through a reproductive cycle, during which they divide to form new cells. DNA is the genetic material—the blueprint—the cell requires for replication, telling cells what to do and how to do it.

When a cell is irradiated, whether through radioactive seeds or external beam radiation, reactive chemicals called free radicals are produced. Free radicals can damage DNA, ultimately interfering with the cell division process.

Radiation damages all cells, both cancerous and non-cancerous. The damage shows up during the reproductive phase of the cell. Cancer cells are their own worst enemy in this regard because they don't follow the rules. They never have. They expand and reproduce as they please, doing so more rapidly than normal cells. Because cancer cells go through faster reproductive cycles than normal cells, they die more quickly from radiation damage than normal cells. In a nutshell, the cancer cell is irradiated, free radicals appear, the DNA in the cell is injured, the cell cannot repair itself and does not divide, and the cancer cell dies.

The prostate gland is an odd and lazy fellow. Its cells, including the cancerous ones, divide more slowly than cells in other organs. Therefore, in the prostate, cancer cells continue dying—unable to replicate—weeks, even months after radiation ends.

What happens to all those exterminated cells? They have an inelegant ending indeed. The end products of metabolic breakdown, they are washed unceremoniously out of the body in urine.

What happens to normal cells during radiation? If the normal cells are close to the cancer being treated, they will receive some radiation and, as a result, some damage. The treating team—doctor, dosimetrist, physicist, and radiation therapist—makes every effort to limit the radiation to areas affected by the cancer. Nevertheless, when the prostate is irradiated, the rectum and bladder will also be irradiated to some degree. Fortunately, normal cells have a greater capacity than their deviant cousins to recover their composure and repair any damage. And the short-term radiation used in therapy is much more damaging to fast-growing cancer cells than it is to slower growing healthy cells. Radiation oncologist Marisa Weiss, M.D., founder of www.breastcancer.org, characterizes the difference between normal and cancerous cells this way:

> "When normal cells are damaged by radiation, they are like a big city with a fire and police department and trained emergency squads to come and 'put out the fire.' Damaged cancer cells are more like a disorganized mob with a bucket."

Monday December 11

7:10 a.m. Dark, dark outside. A hint of light in the heavens, not much more. A legion of crows flying past my window against a dim, overcast sky.

Two days until the radiation therapy begins. Scary to think about, that huge machine hovering over you, your vital organs getting fried. What if they miss their target? But they're extremely careful how they plan and set things up. The BAT machine finds the prostate's exact location every day. They must be good at this. I sincerely hope they're good at this.

Tuesday December 12

Tomorrow is my first radiation treatment. The closer it gets, the more ·I think about it. It seems so final, and one wonders how accurate those beams can be.

It may seem unimportant compared to everything else, but I worry most about an instruction given me at the planning session. "The BAT ultrasound system focuses best on your prostate through a liquid medium," said a radiation therapist. "Therefore we want you to have a full bladder."

A full bladder?

Dr. Bruce has also stressed this. "So that the ultrasound can do its stuff and find your prostate, having a full bladder is helpful."

"Helpful?" I said. "What if I don't?"

"Actually," he said, "it's critical."

I've long had an urgency to urinate as soon as any liquid, even a little, is in my bladder, and now this worries me. How in hell's name will I hold a full bladder for any length of time? Well, tomorrow we'll all find out.

I pray about the radiation. My cousin Ellen tells me I must think it will cure me, and that's the way I'll approach it.

Wednesday December 13

A reprieve. Radiation Oncology calls this morning. "Our equipment is sluggish and Dr. Bruce wants you to come tomorrow."

Sluggish? I don't want the equipment to be sluggish—or anything short of perfect—when it rains its beams of radiation down on me.

I'm a little relieved, though I do want to get this over with. I make an appointment for 3:30 p.m. tomorrow and tell the therapist that's the time I would prefer regularly.

Cold and cloudy, but we haven't had a major storm like those that have raged elsewhere in the country. Something to be grateful for. But winter's far from over.

Thursday December 14

I speak with an old friend who had prostate cancer surgery six years ago. He has mild incontinence, a few drips with exertion. But his major problem is impotence, and it bothers him a lot. He desires sex, but can't get an erection. He's now trying injections 20 minutes before he wants to have sex, but he's not very happy about it.

I begin radiation today. I'm apprehensive, but still believe it will go well. I have confidence in Dr. Bruce and what he says about my having a very good chance of being cured.

In trying to comply with Dr. Bruce's instructions, I drink a lot of water—I mean *a lot* of water—in preparation for going to the hospital, which is about 15 minutes away. My bladder is so full I have to empty it 45 minutes before my 3:30 appointment and again 25 minutes later. I drink a large glass just before leaving home because I am afraid my prostate won't be full enough. I want Dr. Bruce to have a crystal-clear view of my prostate.

Dr. Bruce introduces me to his two radiation therapists, Jill and Bonnie. The department is behind schedule today, and I am taken into the treatment room 20 minutes late—with a *very* full bladder!

Jill holds out a small, white towel. "This your modesty towel," she says. "I'll hold it in front of you, and we'll ask you to lower your pants a bit so we can see the crosshatches."

She holds the towel in front of my pubic area, and I slide my pants and underwear down partway. Then I take the towel and hold it in front of me as I lie down on the table. The therapists pull my pants down a little farther, then place my legs and feet in the mold fabricated a couple of weeks earlier to keep me still and in proper position.

Just suffering with a brimming bladder isn't enough.

"I'm going to press down with this," Bonnie says, lifting a probe from the BAT ultrasound machine, which stands ominously beside the table. "It might be a little uncomfortable, but it helps us see the prostate."

Placing the probe over one side of my bladder, she pushes down—hard—for about five seconds. She lets up and moves the probe to the other side of my bladder and again pushes down hard. Then, she repeats the process three or four times.

Okay, I think, if I lose it, I lose it. I'll just fill it up again and we'll start over. I pray fervently.

Imagine lying on a hard table with a distended bladder and having somebody lean on it with an elbow. That's pretty much what this feels like.

I can't see the ultrasound screen, but I can tell by the therapists' remarks that the bladder and prostate are—hallelujah—visible.

Dr. Bruce arrives and looks at the screen. "Dr. Priest has overdone the bladder a little bit today. Tomorrow the prostate's position will be different." He has previously explained to me that the prostate can move up to 1-1/2 centimeters from day to day depending on what's in the rectum and bladder.

Finally a hydraulic lift raises the table so that I'm be closer to the huge machine hovering over me. After seeing to it that I am positioned properly and explaining to me what will happen next, everyone vacates the room, leaving me alone.

Soon there is an odd vibratory sound that lasts 10 to 12 seconds. I later learn that the sound means that radiation is being delivered. When the sound stops, the machine rotates to a new position. The sound begins again, then stops; the machine rotates again; and eventually I receive radiation from six different directions.

The ceiling in the bone scan room where I'd had my first X-rays had been blank. But the ceiling here is covered with pictures, beautiful sunlit forest scenes. And there is enough room that I don't feel claustrophobic.

I can't sense the radiation at all. Just my bladder, which feels like it's going to burst.

When the treatment is over, the therapists come in, lower the table, and help me up. I leave the room, pushing past Dr. Bruce and declaring, "I'm going to the bathroom."

I do, expelling a plentiful quantity of urine. Without question, it is the fullest my bladder has been in years.

But it's over. And now I know what I'm up against. The bladder thing will be annoying, but even if it's as full as it was today, I can tolerate it. I hope I won't fill it quite so much the next time. But, judging by today's events, achieving a happy medium is not an exact science.

I see Dr. Bruce again. "Are there any foods or drinks I should avoid?"

"For now, no," he says. "Eat what you want and we'll see how things go. There was a report that vitamin C can reduce the effect of what the radiation's trying to do, kill cancer cells. I don't think that's been corroborated."

I asked Jill, the therapist, about radiation fatigue.

"It comes on during the last couple of days of the week in the latter weeks of treatment," she says. "Patients like you having only a small, highly targeted area treated might not feel much at all."

We'll see. I hope she's right.

Brachytherapy (Radioactive Seeds)
for Prostate Cancer

Placing radioactivity in or near a targeted area, frequently a tumor, is called brachytherapy. To treat prostate cancer this way, tiny radioactive seeds are implanted in the prostate gland to impart concentrated, localized radiation. The seeds are metal-encapsulated pellets containing the radioisotope Iodine-125 or Palladium-103. A seed is about 1/8th of an inch long and has the thickness of a paper clip.

Seed implantation for prostate cancer has been done for over 20 years. Though permanently implanted, the seeds are sources of decreasing radioactivity. Iodine-125 has a half-life of 60 days and Palladium-103 a half-life of 17 days, which means that Iodine-125 loses half of its radioactivity every 60 days, while Palladium-103 loses half of its radioactivity every 17 days. No significant differences in clinical outcomes have been seen between the two isotopes, in terms of either success rates or rates of complications.

Brachytherapy is generally performed in cases where the prostate cancer is localized (that is, the cancer has not metastasized, or spread, beyond the prostate) and the patient has a PSA of 10 or less and a Gleason score of 7 or less. Like most procedures, brachytherapy is done slightly differently by different physicians in different hospitals in different parts of the country. Brachytherapy can be used in combination with external beam radiation.

After planning carefully with a computer, and using a template for seed placement, seeds are implanted in the prostate gland during an outpatient procedure under general or spinal anesthesia. The patient usually goes home the same day, sometimes with a catheter in place. The number of seeds used in the procedure can vary from 50 to 100.

Complications from permanent seed implants can be consequential. Radiation-induced impotence may develop over time and is reported to occur in about 25 percent of all patients. Incontinence, however, is much rarer, occurring in around 1 percent of patients who undergo the treatment.

Other urinary symptoms, such as pain or difficulty urinating, increased frequency, and decreased urinary stream, occur in about 30 percent of patients, but these numbers could improve with newer techniques, such as peripheral loading of seeds to reduce radiation to the urethra. These urinary symptoms tend to dissipate over time, but they can last a year or longer. Four to 5 percent of patients may require surgical intervention for urinary obstruction. Rectal complications, such as burning, pain, and diarrhea, occur in less than 5 percent of patients.

After the procedure, some precautions are advisable to avoid radiating other persons. For the first 4 to 8 weeks after brachytherapy, children shouldn't sit on the patient's lap, and there should be no prolonged close contact with pregnant women and people under 45 years of age. Sexual intercourse may be resumed after two weeks, but a condom should be used for the first two months. Instructions to patients after prostate cancer seeding will vary depending upon the risk of radiation exposure and the particular practices of the institution where the procedure is performed. Always follow the specific instructions that your health care provider gives you.

The bottom line is this: prostate cancer patients with a PSA of 0 to 10 have almost identical cancer-free results after eight to nine years whether they have brachytherapy (radioactive seeds), prostatectomy (surgery), or external beam radiation.

Friday December 15

I tell several people about my treatment and bladder situation. They sympathize. One says, "A pregnant woman must have a full bladder for an ultrasound test. My wife did, and it was darn uncomfortable."

Another says, "Once, while I was skiing, my bladder got full. I had to take a chairlift to get to the chalet and got on the wrong one. Finally I took the right one, and at the top got my skis off and walked 100 yards to the bathroom. I was ready to kill anyone ahead of me."

Today's treatment goes much more smoothly. It is quicker, my bladder is not as full, and the therapists are happy with the results.

The PSA in my blood after my first treatment measures 6.28. Not good. It's gone up. I talk with one of Dr. Bruce's associates.

"There's nothing at all to be alarmed about," he says. "It could be coming from prostatitis."

While picking up a new pair of eyeglasses at the optician's, I see an old friend and tell her I am in treatment for you-know-what. Another friend also comes by. I used to work with both of them, and we have a nice reunion right there in the waiting room.

Saturday December 16

Exactly 4:00 a.m. A fair amount of snow tonight—a beautiful winter wonderland. I feel pretty good about my cancer treatment. I hope my PSA goes down next time, but all kinds of therapies are available if I need them.

Sunday December 17

We go to a party. I mention that I have prostate cancer.

"Get it out," someone says. "I had surgery on mine."

The man who had surgery and now wears diapers is also here.

Monday December 18

I'm getting this bladder thing down to a science. Before the last two radiation treatments, I emptied my bladder two hours ahead of time, then drank half a glass of water, and my bladder was fine both times.

As I sign in at the Radiation Oncology waiting room, a television camera monitors me from directly above. In an adjoining room, the therapists can read the sign-in page on a television monitor.

"It's the best way we've found to know who's arrived and get them into the treatment room," Dr. Bruce tells me.

I feel nothing during radiation. I simply lie still and pray.

Tuesday December 19

Sunny day. I empty my bladder at 1:30, then drink a small amount of water, and my bladder feels full even before I leave the house for my 3:30 treatment. Maybe I don't have this figured out after all.

Every day the therapist presses down on the bladder with the probe to see where the prostate is. I don't mind. I want her to know precisely where it is before bombarding me with radiation.

Wednesday December 20

I empty my bladder at noon and don't drink afterwards, and my bladder is full when I get to Radiation. Clearly, this bladder stuff is not an exact science.

I've never been able to tell when the radiation is on and when it is off, so I ask Bonnie about this now: "Is the radiation on when the machine's rotating?"

"No," says Bonnie, "it comes on when it's stationary and makes sort of a funny sound."

"Oh, okay, I know the sound."

Of course now that I know when the radiation is on, the first moment I hear the sound I tense up and involuntarily contract my urethral sphincter, the ring-shaped muscle controlling urine flow.

Don't ask me why it happens, but it does and I can't stop it. I worry that the contraction momentarily changes the prostate's position.

I ask Dr. Bruce about this. He looks a little surprised. I don't think anyone's asked him this before. They just lie still and take their treatment.

"I don't think it would change anything," he says.

Five treatments down, many more to go.

Thursday December 21

The shortest day of the year. The sun is at its lowest in the sky. I have my baseball cap in place.

I like the sun when it's out, even for these brief hours. I don't mind wearing the cap.

When I get to the hospital, Jill approaches me. "We're having trouble with the radiation machine. It's been working all day, but stopped just before you arrived."

The therapists are about to give me the day off when the repairman walks in. Within minutes they are ready for me.

The BAT machine is also on the fritz, and I worry about this, but Dr. Bruce elects to go ahead with the treatment. Most men have received radiation treatment without its being guided by a BAT machine, I reason, and the complication rate is low, very low. So I shouldn't worry about it. And I won't.

Friday December 22

I have my seventh treatment. The department is a little behind schedule, and a mailman in uniform goes in before me.

"You won't have to breech medical privacy," I tell Bonnie, who is escorting me into the treatment room, "and tell me what disease the mailman's being treated for. I already know. When he came out, he hightailed it for the bathroom."

She laughs.

Jill mentions the X-rays taken after yesterday's therapy. "They tell us that the radiation's going exactly where we want," says Jill.

"Fine with me," I say.

I play tennis with friends. Halfway through the match, the tape covering one of the crosshatches on my skin falls off onto the court. I guess Sally is wrong about how secure the tape is.

I pick it up, show it to the guys, and tell them what it is for.

"Ooh," says Craig, turning away, "that's pretty gruesome."

Saturday December 23

Still no obvious effects from the radiation. I am very active today, shopping and driving around with my wife. As I write this we await our son Eric, motoring home from Chicago with three friends, all staying here over Christmas and New Years.

Monday December 25

Christmas Day, and we have a full house. Our son David stops here on his way back from Asia and brings flowered leis from Hawaii for everyone. In the evening he leaves, but the Chicago gang stays on.

One of the group is an artist, and after Christmas dinner Ilka takes him to her small study overlooking the lake.

"Paint something for me," she says, gesturing toward the walls and ceiling.

"How about a tree?" he asks.

"A tree? Fine. I'll get the paint."

He mixes several colors of house paint and within six hours has rendered a remarkably vivid tree from floor to ceiling—trunk, branches, leaves and all, covering the space's interior. It's wonderful, and Ilka adores it.

"You'd never have had this had I not developed prostate cancer," I tell her. "We'd have been out of here, celebrating Christmas in Florida."

Radical Prostatectomy:
Surgical Removal of the Prostate Gland

Urologists tend to believe that surgery is the best way to treat prostate cancer, and many recommend radical prostatectomy for the disease. A brief description of the "nerve-sparing" form of the surgery follows.

The surgeon approaches the prostate gland through an incision in the abdomen. The urethra, a tube that passes through the prostate as it carries urine from the bladder, is severed immediately below the prostate gland. If the nerves that are responsible for erections are not affected by the cancer, they are spared. But sparing the nerves requires great skill, since these nerves run so close to the wall of the prostate. The cancerous prostate gland is cut away from the bladder and removed, and the urinary passageway is rebuilt by sewing the urethra to the bladder.

If this sounds simple, it isn't.

In his book *Dr. Patrick Walsh's Guide to Surviving Prostate Cancer*, Dr. Walsh, who invented and perfected the nerve-sparing surgery, writes that "radical prostatectomy is a tricky operation, one of the most difficult in medicine. There can be tremendous, at times life-threatening, blood loss."

Radical prostatectomy is a difficult operation because bleeding can sometimes make it hard for the surgeon to see. It is also difficult because the surgeon is working in a tight space surrounded by fragile organs that are susceptible to injury. And it is difficult because the surgeon must avoid damaging the two tiny nerve bundles controlling erections.

Cutting the urethra is a delicate procedure because if the cut is too near the prostate, cancer cells might be left in surrounding tissue. If the cut is too far from the prostate, the urethral sphincter (the muscular ring that tightens and relaxes to control the flow of urine) can be injured, which might lead to incontinence. According to Dr. Walsh, "the surgical line here is literally not much more than a hairbreadth."

Because radical prostatectomy is a difficult operation, the surgeon's experience and ability are vital to a successful outcome. In a study in the January 2000 issue of the journal *Urology,* Dr. Walsh and his co-authors point out that the procedure has far better results when performed at a center of excellence by a surgeon who does them in large numbers. Doctors at other centers reported that one year after surgery only 50 percent of their patients were continent and only 10 to 30 percent were potent. These figures are in marked contrast to those from centers of excellence, where up to 93 percent of patients reported being continent and 65 percent reported being potent.

Complications from radical prostatectomy can include blood loss, infection, urinary incontinence, impotence, even death. According to the American Foundation for Urologic Disease, about 1 in every 200 to 400 men who have the operation die from complications such as heart attacks and blood clots. Dr. Walsh, however, reports that in a Johns Hopkins study of over 2,800 patients, only 3 died.

Tuesday December 26

Three days off radiation because of the holiday. Back to it today. The therapists apply new tape over the crosshatch.

Dr. Bruce is in the treatment room almost every day checking things out before the radiation begins. I see him in the office after today's session.

"How are you doing?" he asks.

"I have to work a little harder than usual emptying my bladder," I say.

"That could be from radiation."

"I don't seem to have any other side effects."

He smiles. "I think we have a very good patient here."

Wednesday December 27

Ninth treatment, and all is well. I drink water at the club at 1:30 before a 3:30 treatment, then twice again at home.

When I urinate immediately after my treatment, there doesn't seem to be much urine. I see Bonnie in the hallway.

"Was there enough urine in my bladder?" I ask. "Didn't seem like much when I emptied it."

"It was full enough," she says. "Radiation irritates the bladder. Just now perhaps you couldn't empty it completely."

This suggestion surprises me, but maybe she's right.

Ilka and I enjoy dinner with friends, then go to a play. It is one of the best dinners we've ever had, but one of the worst stage events we've ever seen.

I ask for an aisle seat, not because the play is bad and I want to get away, but because after what Bonnie has said I'm not sure how my bladder will act. It turns out not to be a problem. I still have no radiation fatigue.

Thursday December 28

Bonnie says that the radiation is irritating my bladder. I hope it's also "irritating" the hell out of my prostate.

Today I take a minidisk player with me and listen to music with earphones during treatment. I'm hoping to mask the sound of the radiation machine, despite Dr. Bruce's belief that my momentary sphincter contractions won't affect the position of the prostate. "Actually, I think they might," my brother Jack had said when I asked him about it. "Why don't you listen to music? But make it something you don't like, because in the future you'll probably associate that music with bad memories."

I don't want to risk contracting my prostate out of position, so I take my brother's advice. When the music is turned on, I can't tell whether the radiation is on or off, and so—no contractions

"Can you make it in early tomorrow," asks Jill, "so the staff can get away for the New Year's holiday?"

"Sure," I say.

My 10th treatment today, almost one-quarter done.

Friday December 29

Snowy driving, but I make it to therapy. Afterwards I get stuck in snow in the driveway at home. Ilka and I shovel for a long while and I wonder whether radiation fatigue might be coming on.

Monday January 1

No treatment over the long holiday weekend. A little bladder and rectal irritation—nothing bad, just a bit more urgency to go.

Tuesday January 2

The therapists weigh me before treatment. I haven't lost any weight, although it isn't uncommon to lose one or two pounds a week during radiation therapy.

I learn something reassuring today.

"What if a patient's bladder isn't full enough?" I ask Bonnie as she escorts me in.

"Not a problem," she says. "We send you out to the waiting room for a cup of water and wait until it is."

This is good news. I don't have to be so nervous about filling my bladder or keeping it full. Yes, it's better if it's full, but the therapy won't be compromised if it isn't.

The radiation treatment as usual takes just minutes. Afterwards I see Dr. Bruce in an examining room.

"How are you feeling?" he asks.

"I have a little urgency of bowel and bladder," I say, "but no sexual dysfunction or fatigue."

He pauses. "A new publication just came out confirming that 3D-CRT is as good as or better than seeds for prostate cancer."

"This confirms my conclusion that external beam radiation will be the norm for this disease in the future."

He nods. "But urologists are hardly convinced."

Once again, I am glad that I've taken time to research all the possible treatments for this condition.

Wednesday January 3

A therapist I have seen only once before does the ultrasound, pressing more heavily over the pubic bone with the probe than anyone has done previously. It is painful.

Later I mention this to Bonnie. "That's where your bladder was today. That's why we use this," she says, putting a hand on the BAT machine.

Thursday January 4

I overfill my bladder, and, in the Murphy's Law world of modern medicine, Radiation is running late when I arrive. Part of the reason that the therapists are off schedule is that a small boy has had to be brought in for treatment on an emergency basis. He is seven or eight years old, and my paltry problems, I tell myself as I pace the waiting room, pale in comparison to what he and his family must be going through.

Different therapists today, and I tell them they will have no trouble finding my bladder. "It was full," one says afterwards.

Walking the dogs I meet a neighbor on the sidewalk. He's a retired physician and I mention that I have prostate cancer.

"I had it too," he says, "and it was treated surgically." He's the third neighbor within a few houses who's had prostate cancer surgery. "Had it 10 years ago—by the head of urology at the university—and was it an ordeal! My prostate was large and the disease was advanced. I was in the operating room from 7:30 in the morning till 3:00 in the afternoon. My blood count fell to 7, and they gave me three units of blood. I was in the hospital for a month."

He's okay now and disease-free. But I'll bet he's incontinent, and chances are high that he's impotent.

He says something else disconcerting. "If you biopsied every prostate gland, you'd find abnormal cells in each gland which under a microscope could be construed as cancer."

I remember asking my urologist how he knew that the biopsy specimen labeled as mine was actually mine, not someone else's. If you believe what my neighbor says, it doesn't matter. Every man has prostate cancer, and I'm one of the lucky ones, treating it before it becomes bad—invasive, painful, life-threatening—rather than just letting it stew there as it does in every male.

Dr. Bruce has told me that prostate cancer's natural history isn't well understood.

Hormonal Treatment for Prostate Cancer

Hormonal therapy for prostate cancer is a complex and somewhat controversial topic. In general, hormone treatment is used to inhibit prostate cancer, prolong survival, and improve lifestyle. It can shrink tumors and ease such symptoms as bone pain, fatigue, and difficulty urinating.

Hormonal therapy is not a cure for prostate cancer, and it can cause significant side-effects, such as hot flashes and impotence. Men who have untreated cancer that is confined to the prostate and are good candidates for surgery or radiation may want to consider those options over hormonal treatment.

Hormone therapy is commonly used in the following situations:

- when cancer has spread beyond the prostate gland to nearby tissues or other parts of the body

- when the patient has had radiation or surgery and the cancer has returned

- to reduce pain from tumors which have spread (usually to bone)

- to shrink an enlarged prostate before other treatment is undertaken (seed therapy, external beam radiation, cryotherapy, or surgery) in order to increase the chances that the treatment will work

- before, during, and after radiation of some tumors

How do hormones help treat prostate cancer? Prostate cancer cells are driven to proliferate and flourish by the dominant male hormone, testosterone. If the level of this hormone in the body is reduced, the cancer cells become sluggish. But not forever. Over the next one to five years, the cancer cells adapt to the reduced male hormone level and begin expanding and spreading again.

How is testosterone reduced? Administering estrogen, a female hormone, was once the most common approach to reducing levels of testosterone in prostate cancer patients. But this practice has declined due to the potential for such serious complications as heart disease, blood clots, and stroke.

Most testosterone (90 to 95 percent) is produced in the testicles. The most direct way to decrease this hormone is by surgically removing the testicles (an operation called "orchiectomy"). A relatively uncomplicated procedure, it can be done in an outpatient setting.

Testosterone production from the testicles can also be reduced by administering drugs, an approach now preferred to orchiectomy. The most common of these drugs are the luteinizing hormone-releasing hormone analogs (LHRH)—known by the brand names Lupron and Zoladex—which are given by injection every one to four months. If a man has advanced cancer and chooses to have an LHRH drug, it may be administered indefinitely.

Some testosterone (about 5 to 10 percent of the total) is produced elsewhere in the body, mostly by the adrenal glands. If an anti-androgen drug is given along with an LHRH analog, testosterone production can be stopped completely. Experts do not agree whether doing this yields better treatment for prostate cancer than either LHRH analogs or orchiectomy by themselves.

Friday January 5

I sometimes have premonitions. Today I am inexplicably nervous before treatment. And it turns out with good reason.

I sit for 10 minutes in the waiting room, then Jill walks me in for treatment. "We're taking reference ultrasound pictures today," she says, "but it won't take longer than usual."

Famous last words. To get the pictures, they push harder and longer on my bladder than ever before, and unfortunately it is very full—second in fullness only to that first day.

When they are through, the radiation begins. But the machine isn't acting normally. It remains in each stationary position for much longer than usual, as if stuck. What a relief when it begins rotating again!

I don't know what is going on. The therapists try to explain it to me over an intercom, but with the music in my ears I can't understand a word they say. I don't want to move to turn the disk player off, because I don't know when the radiation is on.

Finally the therapists come in. "We were having technical difficulty," says Jill, helping me off the table. "We've had to direct the machine manually, and that's what took so long."

I have been on the table for 35 minutes, long enough to hear 11 songs by the singing group America. Not a pleasant experience.

But—whew!—it's over. I hope I have no more premonitions.

> This incident turned out to be the least pleasant experience I had during radiation therapy. But compared to surgery, not so terrible at all.

Saturday January 6

Holiday reception and dinner at a neighbor's home. Two of the older attendees have undergone prostatectomies. Three, including our host. Surgery was clearly the preferred treatment when their cancers were discovered. Actually, it's still the preferred treatment.

Monday January 8

I am not as nervous about treatment today. Last time, after things didn't go so well, I jokingly told Jill, "I hope the machine will be fixed by Monday."

She took me seriously, and today introduces me to the department physicist, Dr. Payne. "The machine's gotten out of tune," he says. "But that doesn't affect the radiation delivered to the patient. It means the machine doesn't like it when it's told to rotate automatically to the next field. The therapists have to direct it manually."

Okay, no problem, as long as I know what's going on. Today's treatment goes slowly but uneventfully, the machine being controlled manually, and that's that.

Tonight for some reason I have a feeling of exhilaration. I don't know why.

Tuesday January 9

I get lucky with the bladder. Forty minutes before treatment it is so full that I empty it. Then, worried that it won't be full enough, I drink a fair amount of water.

The therapists are really backed up today, and while sitting in the waiting room I look around at the other patients. Among them are a short woman who uses crutches and drags one foot as she walks, a seven- or eight-year-old boy with his younger sister and parents, an elderly man, and a young soldier in a camouflage uniform whose hair is short, thin and frizzy as if he's been receiving chemotherapy. Cancer knows no boundaries.

I don't go in until almost an hour after the scheduled time. By then there's plenty of urine in my bladder.

I'm nearly 40 percent through with the treatments.

A phone call from Mary and Don. "A few days ago," he says, "I was diagnosed with prostate cancer. We heard you recently were, too."

"Come on over tomorrow," I say, "and we'll talk about it."

Wednesday January 10

Don and Mary arrive, and Ilka and I talk with them in my study for almost two hours about various aspects of prostate cancer. They are most interested in how I arrived at my decision. Having met with their urologist the day before, they are amazed when I describe the high complication rates for radical prostatectomy.

"He didn't tell us that," she says. "He mentioned incontinence and impotence as possibilities, but didn't go into them in much detail and said that for impotence they have Viagra and pumps. We had no idea that complications occur that frequently."

"That's why it's good to look into this for yourself," I say.

She looks at Don, then me. "You're a doctor and you've done all this research. Your conclusions sound pretty good to me."

Don agrees.

I refer them to Dr. Bruce.

Thursday January 11

Another treatment, but none tomorrow, as they plan to work on the equipment. The machine is still turning slowly.

I see Dr. Bruce. "I haven't had skin irritation," I say.

"You won't get that," he says. "We administer the radiation from several angles, and therefore each skin area gets a lesser dose."

"I haven't had fatigue."

"You will get that, I'm afraid."

Friday January 12

A day off radiation (and bladder control) while they work on the equipment at the hospital. Having a day off feels good.

Monday January 15

The machine is repaired, so today it rotates automatically. It's two to three times faster when it works this way. As usual, I listen to Bach and pray.

Tuesday January 16

The 21st of 42 treatments. I'm halfway home. Smooth therapy, the machine operating perfectly.

"I've felt no fatigue," I tell Bonnie. "Is that normal when you're halfway through treatment?"

Her answer disappoints me. "Yes, that's common."

I'm hoping the BAT system, which permits extremely accurate targeting, will cut down on the chance of radiation-induced fatigue. But Dr. Bruce says I'll get it anyway.

"Don was in today," Dr. Bruce says. "Thanks for referring him."

"I'm keeping a journal of all this," I say.

"A very good idea," he says. "Information about prostate cancer is sorely lacking to the general public. You should publish it because you're a physician and a writer."

"And a patient."

"It would provide a great service."

"I've completed 21 of 42 treatments."

He chuckles. "All patients keep track of how far along they are."

Don calls tonight. "We're going to Florida for eight days to think it over, but I'm 90 percent sure I'll choose radiation. Thanks for talking to us."

"I should publish this journal," I tell Ilka after hanging up, "to give patients another perspective. But urologists would hate me."

Cryotherapy (Freezing) for Prostate Cancer

Hoping to join surgery, radioactive seeds, and external beam radiation as a mainstream treatment for prostate cancer, cryotherapy is the new kid on the block. While about 190,000 new cases of prostate cancer were diagnosed in the United States in 2001, only 3,000 patients underwent cryotherapy.

Less is known about the effectiveness of cryotherapy compared to the three more common treatments for prostate cancer. Yet cryotherapy is not a new idea. Cryoablation (freezing) of the prostate gland was first done in the 1960s and 1970s, but the lack of adequate monitoring of the freezing process led to major complications, and the procedure was abandoned. With improvements in technology, cryosurgery emerged again in the 1980s and has gradually progressed from an experimental technique to a viable alternative therapy for prostate cancer. One seven-year study of cryotherapy as the primary treatment for prostate cancer found that targeted cryoablation equaled or surpassed the outcomes achieved by external beam radiation and seeds.

Cryosurgery may be used as the primary treatment of early localized and locally advanced tumors, and for recurring cancer in the gland after external beam radiation or seeds have failed. If the prostate is large, the gland might be need to be shrunk using hormonal therapy prior to the procedure.

Cryotherapy is performed in a manner similar to seed implantation. The patient may go home the same day or the following day, and resume normal activities within a few days.

Prior to doing the procedure, a 3-D computer image of the prostate may be generated to aid the physician in planning where to place the needles, or cryoprobes. As in seed therapy, a template is prepared through which needles or probes are passed before entering the prostate.

The procedure is performed with an ultrasound probe inserted into the rectum, giving the operators an accurate image of what is happening. With the needles or probes positioned in the prostate, high-pressure argon gas or liquid nitrogen causes the probes to freeze, which in turn causes balls of ice to form within the gland. The balls increase in size and coalesce, filling and freezing the entire gland and a margin of tissue surrounding it. The operators allow the ice balls to form, then thaw, and then use the needles or probes to carry out one or more additional freezing and thawing cycles. Ice crystals form within the prostate cells, both cancerous and healthy, and the cells die.

To avoid freezing the urethra, which runs through the prostate gland, warm water is circulated through a catheter inserted into the penis. After the procedure, white blood cells begin to clear away the dead prostate cells, and the gland is eventually replaced by scar tissue.

There is a scarcity of good long-term data on prostate cryotherapy, but early results suggest that there are both advantages and disadvantages to the procedure.

Among the advantages: If necessary, cryotherapy can be repeated, while surgery and external beam radiation cannot. Cryosurgery has a shorter recovery time than the other treatments. Rates of incontinence appear to be low (only 4 percent in the best study to date). And patients who suffer a recurrence of their cancer after treatment with radiation, whether external beam or seeds, can be treated with cryoablation.

The disadvantages? While incontinence is infrequent, the impotency rate is high. The nerves controlling erections lie adjacent to the sides of the prostate and are usually frozen when the gland is frozen. Most men experience erectile dysfunction after cryoablation. But a recent study from the University of Calgary, reported in the June 2002 issue of the journal *Urology*, found that about half those with impotence had recovered sexual function after three years. Work is also being done on freezing techniques that preserve the nerves.

Generally, rates of complications from cryotherapy are low. However, if cryotherapy is used to treat patients whose radiation therapy has failed, complication rates can rise significantly. These complications can include incontinence, a fistula (or hole) between the rectum and urethra, pelvic pain, and injury to the urethra. For patients whose recurrent post-radiation tumor is large, cryoablation may not be a suitable option.

As with other surgical procedures, including radical prostatectomy, results depend at least partly on the skill of the surgeon. Not every urologist does cryotherapy. Those who do are found by word of mouth, referral, and searching on the Internet.

Friends drop off the May 29, 2000, issue of *New Yorker* magazine. It contains a long article on prostate cancer by a medical oncologist, Jerome Groopman, titled "The Prostate Paradox." I read it aloud to Ilka. The writer has interviewed several physicians who treat the disease variously with surgery, seeds and external beam radiation. As usual, there is no clear-cut favorite. The patient must choose for himself.

A urologist is the first physician to talk with a patient after a biopsy. Having done the procedure, the urologist presents the results, telling the patient he has cancer. Thus the urologist has the first shot at advising the patient what to do. Most urologists recommend radical prostatectomy. When the average man hears the word "cancer," he wants it out of his body as soon as possible. Is it any wonder he follows his doctor's advice to have surgery?

Wednesday January 17

Treatment 22 of 42. Dr. Bruce stops to talk to me while I am in the waiting room. He's going to Arizona tomorrow for a short vacation.

I feel tired this afternoon, but play tennis anyway. Maybe a little fatigue?

My appetite isn't great, but I haven't lost much weight—at most, a pound or two. The therapists weigh me once a week. I have some irritation of bladder and bowel, more urgency than usual. Dr. Bruce says this will disappear after the treatment ends.

As he advised, I eat and drink whatever I want. But based on the what he said, I'm staying away from vitamin C.

Thursday January 18

Treatment goes about as smoothly as possible today. The therapists are ready for me two minutes after I arrive, and the machine rotates quickly. I am in the radiation room just six or seven minutes.

Jill and Bonnie are helpful as always. I'm probably the only one of their patients who listens to music. They make sure my minidisk player doesn't fall off the table while I'm climbing onto it.

"What do you listen to?" asks Jill, fingering the player.

"A Bach Brandenburg Concerto," I say, "but which one I don't know. I always listen to the same one because the volume remains relatively constant throughout. If the music has quiet passages, I hear the radiation start, which I don't want to do."

I've had 23 treatments; I'm on the downslope now. The finish line's still way out there, but at least it's in sight.

I'm less nervous about the treatment now. Why should I be nervous at all? Well, a beam of lethal energy is entering my body. I must lie still so it doesn't fry something it's not supposed to, and I have to do this with an uncomfortably full bladder.

But these are minor inconveniences compared to incontinence and impotence. Not being able to hold your urine is a damn nuisance. I wouldn't want to contend with it. Sexual dysfunction can be a big deal for a man—no matter how old he is—to say nothing of his partner. The *New Yorker* article said men never stop thinking about sex.

Friday January 19

Treatment again goes very smoothly. I still can't say I've felt fatigue, though I'm 57 percent through with radiation. The urgencies of bladder and bowel continue, and Dr. Bruce says they'll get worse as treatment proceeds.

Saturday January 20

I might have radiation fatigue this morning. I get up at 7:10 and feel like going back to bed, which is very unusual for me. I lie down on the couch in my study and rest for two hours.

Sunday January 21

I get up at 6:00 this morning, work on a revision of my second book for a couple of hours, then go back to bed for a nap.

When I get up again I have trouble urinating. The urine dribbles out, and my bladder doesn't fully empty. Urethral strictures and benign prostatic hyperplasia cause the same thing. With me it's radiation-induced and will go back to normal when the treatment's over.

Monday January 22

Our son David's 33rd birthday. We have guests for lunch, and I drink water and coffee. I don't empty my bladder afterwards. It is too full when I go to therapy and I have to wait 20 minutes to go in. Otherwise the treatment goes without incident.

> Benign prostatic hyperplasia, or BPH, is swelling or enlargement of the prostate gland. BPH, which is noncancerous, commonly develops in men as they age and can create an urge to urinate while at the same time making urination difficult.

Tuesday January 23

Therapy goes as well. The therapists are waiting for me, my bladder is at the right fullness, and the machine functions properly.

I see Dr. Bruce in an examining room. "Up until now, in case your cancer has spread to the seminal vesicles, we've been radiating them in addition to the prostate," he says. "After two more treatments we'll reduce the field size so the vesicles' superior portions aren't radiated. We don't think they need as much radiation as the prostate."

What Is Watchful Waiting?

"Watchful waiting" means that a diagnosis of prostate cancer has been established, but no treatment has been initiated. The patient simply chooses to wait and watch how the disease progresses. To monitor the progress of the cancer, the patient may periodically have digital rectal exams, PSA tests, transrectal ultrasound, and biopsies.

Watchful waiting is the approach generally followed when a diagnosis of prostate cancer is made in a patient who is 65 to 70 years old or older and who is likely to die from an unrelated condition, such as heart disease, before his prostate cancer becomes problematic. Watchful waiting is also the avenue of choice for men of any age with a short life-expectancy or a serious medical problem of another type.

Some patients and physicians believe that too many men with low-grade prostate cancers undergo radical treatment, such as surgery or radiation, that can leave them with far worse conditions (impotence and incontinence) than their slow-growing prostate tumors would ever cause. For patients with small tumors, low Gleason scores, and low PSA levels, watchful waiting is a reasonable option.

Watchful waiting is the most common approach to prostate cancer used in Sweden, no matter what the patient's age. Screening and radical treatments are seldom done. If the patient becomes symptomatic, hormones may be used to treat the symptoms.

Of course, the cancer can spread while a patient waits. Since prostate cancer is "silent" until it spreads, by the time it is symptomatic it may be too late to administer anything but analgesic (pain control) or hormonal therapy.

"What if—to knock out my cancer—I need more radiation than you're planning to give me?"

"You can't have more," he says. "You'll receive 7,560 rads in total, no more, no less. That's all that's safe for your body. That dosage has proven to be much more successful in treating this cancer than 7000 rads. The 8,100-rad regimen given at some institutions is, in my opinion, highly experimental. Many hospitals still give radiation that's not 3D-CRT and do it without the BAT system. Their accuracy in placing the radiation is not as good, and more side effects occur."

"I feel a little tired today," I say, "but not fatigued."

He smiles. "You've taken good care of yourself, and it's paying off."

The woman on crutches who drags one leg must be finished with her therapy. "I'll miss you all," I hear her tell a therapist on her way back to treatment. I envy her, but I'll be done pretty soon myself.

Tonight a local television station airs a story about prostate cancer radiation, featuring Dr. Bruce and a prostate cancer patient. Dr. Bruce asked me if I wanted to be the patient on TV, but I declined.

Wednesday January 24

After therapy, I ask Bonnie about fatigue. "Would I know it if I had it?"

"You'd feel it," she says. "It's definitely—right there."

Ilka talks at length today with Andrew, an old family friend. "He had prostate cancer treated with radiation by Dr. Bruce," she tells me. "But he experienced prominent fatigue, couldn't do much more than go to treatment and come home and lie on the couch. His PSA now is 0.2 and he feels well."

Thursday January 25

Not long ago, having cancer was a death sentence. Still is in many instances. But the treatments are improving. I'm hopeful about mine.

My appointment is at 3:30 today as usual, but Jill calls at 11:00. "The machine has a glitch. It still produces the type of radiation you receive, but not another kind. Dr. Bruce wonders whether you could come now, because a repairman will be working on it later."

"I'll be there," I say. But I am worried because I've drunk several glasses of water this morning. I empty my bladder, get ready, and go. I am taken right in, the machine functions perfectly, my bladder is fine, and now I have the afternoon off.

Friday January 26

Today the therapists significantly reduce the field they are radiating, by one to one and a half centimeters all around. It still hits my prostate, but little else. I've had rectal and bladder irritation. The reduction might cut down on this.

Don is sitting in the waiting room when I came out of the bathroom (always my destination after treatment). He is here for his planning session. What I presented to him made a difference in what he chose to do.

Monday January 29

Radiation goes well, except that my minidisk player stops working just before the treatment begins. Once or twice I contract my urethral sphincter when the radiation comes on. But a smaller field is being treated now, my contractions are brief, and Dr. Bruce doesn't think it will matter.

"I'm amazed that this far into treatment you've had no fatigue," says Jill. "It's because you came into it in good shape physically and mentally."

"I'm getting used to this bladder stuff," I say. "I might go around with a full bladder even after radiation's over."

She laughs.

This is my 30th treatment. Seventy-one percent through.

Tuesday January 30

Ilka goes with me to therapy just to be along. Things go well except that I've over-filled my bladder.

Thursday February 1

Problems with urinary and bowel urgency and frequency and lots of gas. I have four stools before going to treatment.

I mention my problems to Bonnie, and when I come out of treatment a nurse is waiting. We go into an examination room. "You can take Flomax to reduce the urinary symptoms, and an anti-diarrheal for the bowel," she says. "These symptoms will resolve after your radiation's over, usually in a month, but you'll see a big improvement in the first two weeks."

"I'll go without the medication," I say. "It's not that bad."

Still no noticeable fatigue, now 33 treatments in.

Just off the Radiation Oncology waiting room is the men's room, with which I've become very well acquainted. The only complaint I have about treatment is that the paper towel dispenser in the bathroom shreds the towels as you draw them out, fragments littering the floor. Oh well, if this is the worst thing....

Friday February 2

Two new therapists treat me today, but everything goes smoothly. I have cramping of the rectum, which is somewhat uncomfortable, and urgency of the bladder. Three stools today, four yesterday.

In Dr. Bruce's absence, I see his associate. "I'm not sure that the bowel problem—it's called *tenesmus*—is from radiation," he says. "You might have an intestinal virus."

He gives me a prescription for suppositories, but I don't fill it. Suppositories? The symptoms aren't that bad and, hopefully, won't get to be.

Saturday February 3

Still some rectal irritation, but it seems better today. I ate a low fiber diet yesterday. If I do that more often, the irritation might go away.

"I know several men who've gone to Arizona for a combination of seeds and external beam radiation," says Terry, a friend who also happens to be a physician. "Maybe you should talk to the doctor down there."

"A bit late for that," I say. "I've not only started therapy, I've completed 34 of 42 treatments."

Yet his recommendation makes me stop and wonder whether I have made the right choice after all. What if there is a better way?

No, can't worry about this. No matter what treatment you choose, there are always going to be doubts.

A stunning realization: a week from Wednesday I'll be through with treatment! Through with treatment! I phone Todd and tell him. He can't believe it. The therapy has gone so fast. Not long ago, just getting halfway done seemed a huge accomplishment. Now just over a week to go!

I have diarrhea tonight and barely make it to the bathroom.

Sunday February 4

I get the following e-mail from my college roommate. We're frequently very silly with each other. Among other things he calls me Pea and I call him Thaded.

> Pea,
>
> Haven't heard from you for a while. How are you doing?
>
> As promised, because of your advice I went and had blood work done (first time in a long time). They discovered my triglycerides were way too high, and they suggested I speak with you.
>
> Thaded

I respond with this:

> Thaded,
>
> I have frequency and urgency of bowel and bladder, the full Monty. Every man should undergo radiation.
>
> I've had 34 of 42 treatments. What'll I do when it's over?
>
> Pea

I come down with something new today. They warned me about bowel and bladder problems and radiation fatigue, even skin irritation. But nobody told me about radiation euphoria setting in when I realized that—hallelujah!—I've only got a week and a half of radiation treatments left.

If Treatment Fails—What Next?

No treatment for prostate cancer is 100 percent effective, or it would be the only treatment in use. What happens if surgery fails? If brachytherapy (radioactive seeds) fail? If external beam radiation fails?

All three of these therapies require that patients receive periodic PSA tests, often for the rest of their lives. Any rise in the level of PSA in the blood—whether the treatment was surgery, seeds, or beam radiation—is bad news.

An increase in PSA after the surgical removal of the prostate gland means that some prostate cells remain in the patient's body. If the PSA rises slowly, the assumption is that the cancer cells are in the prostate bed, where the gland used to be. This is only an assumption, however, because there is no easy way to biopsy the area to tell for certain. In this situation, the prostate bed may be treated with external beam radiation. If the PSA continues to rise, hormonal therapy may be used, since hormones can keep the cancer in remission and the PSA down for several years. After hormonal therapy, the treatment is palliative—that is, aimed solely at controlling pain and trying to make the patient as comfortable as possible, as opposed to trying to cure the patient.

If the PSA rises rapidly after surgical removal of the prostate, the assumption is that the cancer has spread to lymph nodes, bone, or other organs. Hormones can keep the cancer in remission for several years. After this hormonal therapy, the treatment is once again palliative—pain medication and some external beam radiation where the cancer has spread to the bone. (This type of external beam radiation is strictly palliative, not curative. It is intended only to slow the growth of the cancer and make the patient more comfortable for as long as possible.)

If the PSA rises after brachytherapy (radioactive seeds), hormones may be given, followed by palliative care as required. In some cases, however, salvage brachytherapy or cryotherapy has been performed for failed seed therapy.

If the PSA rises after external beam radiation, hormonal treatment and later palliative treatment may be provided. External beam radiation cannot be repeated because further radiation would damage surrounding tissues such as the rectum and bladder. In some cases, however, brachytherapy or cryotherapy has been done for failed external beam radiation.

Surgery has rarely been done after seeds or external beam radiation because scar tissue forms as a result of the radiation, making surgery difficult. But a recent study suggests that surgery may still be a viable option for some patients.

Cryotherapy (freezing the prostate gland) is a possible treatment for a local recurrence of prostate cancer after treatment with external beam radiation or seeds. In patients with previous radiation, if a recurrent tumor is small, cryotherapy can be done with a complication rate similar to that in patients who have not been radiated. If the recurrent tumor is large, however, the complication rate is high. These complications include incontinence, the formation of a fistula (or hole) between the rectum and urethra, pelvic pain, and injury to the urethra.

According to the American Cancer Society, chemotherapy is sometimes used for prostate cancer. If the disease has spread beyond the prostate gland and hormonal therapy has ceased to be effective, chemotherapy might slow the cancer's expansion and decrease pain. In other words, chemotherapy might be an option for palliative care when all other options have been exhausted. The American Cancer Society also says that many chemotherapy drugs have been shown to affect prostate cancer, and at least one may help men live longer.

Monday February 5

The last couple of days I've been thinking about getting out of here for someplace warm, probably Florida, because it's fairly close to home should something unfavorable happen because of the radiation—what, I don't know.

I empty my bladder just before leaving for treatment, then feverishly drink water. My bladder is fine during treatment. I'm not going to miss this.

I mention to Bonnie that I have radiation euphoria. She laughs. "I've never heard those words used in conjunction," she says. "Sounds to me like an oxymoron."

No fatigue and 83 percent done. No time for fatigue. Too much to do.

Tuesday February 6

The rectal irritation and urgency have really quieted down since I began a low-fiber, low-residue diet. Was it an intestinal virus a few days ago? The urinary urgency is the same as before.

The 36th treatment goes well. I see Dr. Bruce in an examining room afterwards and, as usual, address him as "Dr. Bruce."

"Tom," he says, suggesting I call him by his first name. I prefer "Dr. Bruce" because I want a doctor/patient relationship. Even though we're both physicians and he knows my brother, as far as my disease goes, he's the doctor and I'm the patient.

He examines my skin. "No radiation burn. You've tolerated this treatment well."

"How many prostate patients avoid fatigue?" I ask, proud of myself.

"Five to 10 percent." He chuckles. "We tested the machine and it really is putting out radiation. How has the treatment gone from your perspective: harder than expected? Easier than expected?"

I have to think. "About as expected. The bladder thing isn't fun, and it's a little nerve-racking to lie in the radiation beam. But that's for a very short time."

"I'll be gone next week when you receive your last treatment. You'll see one of the other doctors."

"You forewarned me about bowel and bladder problems and other things, but didn't tell me about something I contracted over the weekend."

He looks perplexed.

"When I realized how close I was to finishing, I came down with radiation euphoria."

He laughs.

At the very beginning of all this, my brother Bob advised, "Look around and find a doctor you have confidence in and get along with, because you'll be seeing an awful lot of him."

He was right, and Dr. Bruce fills the bill. Highly approachable, he's been helpful throughout.

Ilka makes our reservations for Florida. Man, do I look forward to going.

Wednesday February 7

Because of a snowstorm, I go in for treatment earlier than usual and am taken right in.

"We're even ahead of schedule," says Bonnie.

"More radiation euphoria," I say. "Will it never end?"

Cancer is no laughing matter, nor is radiation. But nearing the end of this course of treatment is really making me feel good.

Thursday February 8

During the night I dream about cancer. In my dream the cancer is a long, thin snake-like creature with a couple of different faces on one end. Hiding in a duct or opening in the ceiling, it strikes quickly, attacking unsuspecting people.

In the waiting room at Radiation I watch a man, doubtless another prostate patient, who is unable to hold his urine any longer. He goes into the bathroom, then drinks water like mad after he come out.

Treatment goes well. "No fatigue," I tell Bonnie. "Don't have time for it."

"There you go," she says. "That's the reason."

Thirty-eight treatments down, 4 to go.

Friday February 9

"I can see the finish line," I tell Jill as we enter the therapy room.

"I'm sure you can."

My disk player stops just before the radiation comes on. Of course I have a contraction every time I hear the radiation start and stop.

Monday February 12

"I'm sprinting toward the finish line," I tell Bonnie, "and I'm not tiring. Dr. Bruce says that 5 to 10 percent of those getting prostate radiation don't develop fatigue."

"Closer to 5 than 10," she says. "One in 20."

I'm really doing well then.

Molly and Mort come to our house for dinner. About 8:00 I feel a little tired. Radiation fatigue? Can it finally be happening to me? Perhaps a little.

Tuesday February 13

Second to last treatment. The therapists are behind schedule, and I have to wait 30 minutes. A new male patient goes in before me. He appears to have lost his hair—from chemotherapy?—and is wearing a stocking cap.

I don't feel tired today. Perhaps yesterday's feeling of fatigue was just normal, everyday tiredness.

Wednesday February 14

Valentine's Day and my last day of radiation. A special valentine.

Since last July, I've had surgery on my knee, with all its attendant pre-operative, surgical, and physical therapy appointments; I've had eye doctor appointments, dental appointments, oncology and urology appointments, bone and CT scan appointments, and an urgent care appointment to treat a bee sting; and, of course, as of this afternoon, I've had 42 radiation treatments for prostate cancer. In the last six months I've visited medical personnel over 60 times. Enough!

I'm taking a box of candy and a card for the folks at Radiation Oncology today. The message on the card reads as follows:

> To Dr. Bruce and the entire staff.
>
> Valentine's Day, my last day of treatment. But you'll go on doing good work and making people better. You're the best!

Because of a personal emergency, Bonnie is out of the office for the second day in a row. I am sorry not to see her.

"She wishes you good luck," says Jill. "She wanted to be here."

Today for the first and only time, a single therapist, Susan, conducts the radiation session. Everything goes well. This is the last time I have to worry about filling my bladder and keeping it full to the appointed hour, and I use my favorite bathroom one last time.

Living with Prostate Cancer

I never imagined I'd have cancer. Cancer, I thought, is something that happens to other people, not to me.

When I was told by my physician that I had cancer, I was stunned, and I remained in a state of shock as I shared the news with my loved ones and friends.

With some cancers a patient must decide fairly quickly what sort of treatment to pursue. This is not usually the case with prostate cancer. Prostate cancer tends to grow slowly, so there is time to consider treatment options. And there are several treatment options to consider. If prostate cancer is caught early, the patient has time to decide between these various options.

For me the decision process was agonizing. Surgery is the so-called "gold standard" recommended by the vast majority of urologists (93 percent). Not surprisingly, my urologist advised radical prostatectomy.

But surgery had what I considered to be unacceptably high rates of serious complications. Radioactive seeds, on the other hand, had fewer complications, and external beam radiation fewer yet.

Resolutely I visited two radiation oncologists, and after a month of research and soul-searching, both alone and with my wife, I chose external beam radiation, amazed that an informed man would choose anything else. As I came to my decision, deep fear changed to relief that I'd found a therapy that would kill the cancer, yet leave me with a normal, healthy life.

I began a series of 42 treatments over 8-1/2 weeks. The radiation itself was painless, but there were side effects. My rectum and bladder, being so close to my prostate, were radiated as well, leading to a temporary urgency in my bowel and bladder. Otherwise, I experienced no side effects from the treatment.

Since treatment my PSA has gone downward. During one of my visits to the radiation oncologist, I asked him when he could say I was out of the woods.

"In 15 years," he told me. "We can't call it a cure from prostate cancer until you've lived 15 years after treatment."

"How many years will I be followed for this cancer?" I asked.

"The rest of your life," he said.

No matter what type of prostate cancer treatment you choose, there is always the risk that the cancer will recur. And this thought may not be very far from your consciousness.

Frequently I think of myself as having had cancer. "I had prostate cancer," I'll mention to an acquaintance. Then I stop. I don't know whether I still have it or not. "I mean I have prostate cancer," I'll say, correcting myself. "I won't be out of the woods for 15 years."

I go to an examining room and meet with Dr. Bruce's associate. "Congratulations on finishing," he says. "You tolerated the radiation very well. Your PSA will go down gradually for a while, after that even more gradually."

"Dr. Bruce told me that it would bottom out about a year and a half after treatment," I say.

"Perhaps a year. Come back for a PSA in eight weeks. The bowel and bladder irritation you have now will start lessening in five to seven days and continue getting progressively better."

This sounds fine to me.

"If a scope were placed in your rectum now," he says, "the anterior wall would look an angry red from the radiation."

I am a little surprised. "Is there a chance of it perforating?"

"No danger of that. It'll take a little time, but it will all heal."

When I leave the room, Jill shakes my hand. "Your insurance policy, the radiation, is now in place and you're well covered," she says She hands me a sheet of paper. "Here's something for all your good work, and to remember us by."

It is a graduation diploma:

In honor of your outstanding courage,
tolerance, and determination.
Best wishes to you from
your Radiation Oncology team.

—Jill, Susan, and Bonnie

I am touched by their thoughtfulness, and they in turn are delighted with my Valentine card and the chocolates.

"We put our cards up on the wall," says Susan. "We call it our trophy wall. Yours will go there, too."

She gives me a sheet of discharge information for male patients who've had pelvic radiation. The document discusses fatigue, skin irritation, nausea, pain, diarrhea, bladder irritation, rectal tenderness, and sexual dysfunction. Fortunately, I've suffered few side effects.

I make the last drive home from the hospital, a drive I've made so many times. But at last I'm through.

Each time I drove to treatment I would use a parking permit for spaces reserved right outside Radiation Oncology's door. When I get home, I notice the parking permit lying in the front seat. I pick it up and drop it into the trash. I have used it more than 40 times, but I don't need it anymore. I'm done.

I swagger into the house. The last treatment is over. What a great feeling!

Thursday February 15

Day 1 since the last of my radiation treatments. Climbing into my pajamas last night, I noticed that the crosshatch used to align me for treatment was still on my left hip, but those from the front and right hip were gone.

I am a little worried and call Susan this morning. "We're enjoying your chocolates," she says.

I ask about the missing markers.

"Not to worry," she says. "The one in front is only a midline indicator, and since it was your last treatment I might not have re-marked it. We routinely feel your sternum and use that as the midline. The two crosshatches on your hips were there when I treated you." She laughs. "Lining you up with only one would be pretty hard."

I feel a bit sheepish.

"I probably removed the one on the right with alcohol," she says. "We like to take them off so they won't remind you guys of what you've been through."

Okay, I'm no longer worried. And still no fatigue.

Going to radiation has become so much a part of my everyday life that today, strangely enough, I feel sadness. I enjoyed the people there and am sad to think that I may never see them again—or only briefly when I visit Dr. Bruce.

Isn't this interesting? Both sad and happy that the treatments are over.

Yes, it was inconvenient to have to drive there so often. Yes, it was unpleasant to have to fill my bladder and keep it full through each appointment. Yes, it was nerve-racking to have to lie motionless under an immense machine while deadly rays were shot into my body.

Yet I did it every day for weeks, and now part of me misses it.

Friday February 16

Day 2 since the end of radiation therapy. My urinary frequency and urgency continue but are mild.

On the spur of the moment Mort invites us to his house for dinner.

"Don't have seconds on the seafood pot," Ilka whispers to me. "I was in the kitchen and saw how he made it. But he cooked the hell out of it, so I'm not too worried you'll get sick."

My appetite has been curtailed by the radiation (though I haven't lost weight), but tonight I am hungry again, and I down seconds of Mort's seafood pot with no ill effects.

Saturday February 17

Day 3 since radiation ended. In 10 days we will leave for Florida.

Terry, a physician and friend, says: "Because of your experiences, I'm going to recommend that my prostate cancer patients see a radiation oncologist in addition to a urologist."

Sunday February 18

Day 4. I sleep through the night. Since the beginning of radiation therapy, I've rarely had to get out of bed to urinate at night.

I have a fairly hard stool and some minor bleeding. Urinary urgency and frequency already seem better. Still some, though, and rectal urgency as well. Seems absurd to be so obsessed with my bowels and bladder. Hopefully I won't have to be much longer.

Tuesday February 20

Day 6. Mark and I take Todd out to lunch. Both Mark and Todd are old friends and know what I've been going through. I drink water during lunch and don't feel the need to urinate even after an hour and a half.

"My urinary and bowel symptoms are lessening," I tell them. "I had an uncomfortable bowel episode two weeks ago, for which I saw the doctor, but overall the symptoms have been mild to moderate, more on the mild side."

A week from today—Florida.

Wednesday February 21

Day 7. My last treatment was a week ago today. I'm feeling good, sleeping through the night.

Still some urinary urgency leading to frequency, but not at night. The urgency happens when I'm near a bathroom, part of my old urgency problem. Interesting that I could hold it when I absolutely had to for radiation.

Friday February 23

Day 9. "Just came from a funeral," a friend tells me. "A man who died of prostate cancer at 75. It wasn't diagnosed until recently and was advanced and had spread to bone."

That's the way it was in the old days and, too frequently, still the way it is. Not a pleasant way to go. Sure glad they found mine early.

Erectile Dysfunction (Impotence) Following Prostate Cancer Treatment

Temporary or even permanent impotence can occur as a consequence of any of the conventional treatments for prostate cancer. Knowing this ahead of time can ease the embarrassment and frustration that men often feel.

Why does prostate cancer treatment so often result in erectile dysfunction? Two tiny nerve bundles that control penile erections pass around and directly adjacent to the prostate gland. Whether the treatment is surgery (prostatectomy), radiation (external beam or brachytherapy), or freezing (cryotherapy), these nerves are vulnerable to injury:

- During surgery, if one or both of the nerves are found to be involved with cancer, the surgeon will remove the involved nerve(s) with the diseased gland, and erectile impairment can be immediate. Disruption of the penile blood supply during radical prostatectomy can also be a factor in post-operative impotence.

- With all types of radiation, impairment of erectile function can develop over time as damage to blood vessels and nerves gradually manifests itself. With external beam radiation, damage to erectile tissue can occur.

- In most cases, impairment is immediate with cryotherapy because the nerves tend to be frozen along with the gland.

In addition to complications from cancer treatment, many other factors can contribute to impotence. Vascular disease linked to high blood pressure, diabetes, high cholesterol, and smoking can impair erections, as can the medications prescribed for hypertension, heart disease, and depression. Even being overweight and not getting enough exercise have been shown to lead to erectile impairment.

But impotence is treatable. The oral medications Viagra, Levitra, and Cialis promote erections by increasing blood flow to the penis. Vacuum pumps draw blood into the penis, also producing an erection. Self-injection of medication into the penis with a needle and insertion of a suppository into the opening at the end of the penis can cause erections as well.

There are also surgical procedures for treating erectile dysfunction. A semi-rigid or inflatable implant can be surgically placed in the penis. During radical prostatectomy, nerve grafts can replace nerves injured or excised in the course of the operation. Much rarer is vascular surgery to repair arteries and veins.

Even if erectile dysfunction has a physical source, it can also have deep psychological implications. Impotence can cause an unfortunate scenario to unfold. If a man can't perform sexually, embarrassment and fear may make things worse. The man's partner may feel guilty or isolated. If the couple is not comfortable discussing the matter, the relationship can suffer. But this doesn't have to be the case. A sex counselor can help the couple cope with self-esteem and intimacy problems, and offer techniques to overcome them.

A final caveat: Before beginning any treatment for erectile dysfunction, consult with your physician.

Saturday February 24

Day 10. Ilka and I shovel the sidewalk and driveway. The snow is quite heavy, but I don't tire. The symptoms of urinary urgency are improving.

Sunday February 25

Day 11. More snow, more shoveling. Mild abdominal cramping.

Monday February 26

Day 12. One more doctor's appointment. The afternoon before we are to leave for Florida, I come down with cramps in my lower-left abdomen. Feels like the diverticulitis I had when I saw the urologist. That problem was addressed with the course of antibiotics he gave me in case I had prostatitis.

I phone Dr. Bruce and describe the symptoms. "I don't think it's related to the radiation," he says.

"I haven't had fatigue," I say.

"If you haven't had it by now, you won't get it. You're one of the fortunate ones."

I don't want to get on a plane and travel with abdominal pain. Our son Eric had a horrible experience in a similar situation. He was on an airplane when a kidney stone became symptomatic.

I go to Dr. Kennedy, an internist, and he examines me.

"It's diverticulitis," he says, "and could be treated with a high-fiber diet." He gives me an antibiotic and suggests that I also take a fiber supplement. I'll take it, but not while I'm on the plane. I don't want to risk any side effects. The diverticulitis doesn't seem so bad anyway.

At 7:15 p.m. Ilka and I go to a wake for Jim. Before Thanksgiving dinner, my brother Jack told us that Jim had cancer. He died of the disease at the age of 71.

It is a nice gathering. Several people ask me how I am doing, and I say that I'm doing well.

Jim's cancer was diagnosed after mine. He didn't have much time. I'm hopeful that my cancer has been found and treated in time.

Tuesday February 27

Day 13. I worry about flying because I might have urgency and not be able to make it to the bathroom. But I have no problems on the flight. We leave home at 5:20 a.m. and arrive in warm, sunny Florida at 12:15 p.m.

As I write this at about 5:00 p.m., Ilka is taking a well-earned nap in the bedroom. It's the first time we've been away from home in a couple of years.

We're entitled to a time without illness, injury, or death threatening us. And yet—Jim's wake was just last evening, so the imminence of death is still with us.

Right now I'm hunting for the best place to put the mouse and keyboard for my computer. We're doing fine. I hope, after all we've been through, that this trip will be something to enjoy.

Wednesday February 28

Day 14. I play tennis outdoors for the first time since last summer. It feels good to be in the sun under a blue sky with hazy clouds, hitting balls on a clay court.

Tony runs the tennis desk, and I regale him with the history of my prostate cancer. His dad had it, too.

From a distance Ilka hears me talking about it. "I've heard enough about that," she calls. "I'm staying away."

"How many times have you heard it?" calls Tony.

"A hundred!" she says.

Thursday March 1

Day 15. Had abdominal pain a couple of days ago. Have been eating a high-fiber diet since and am feeling better.

I talk with a dentist from Minnesota about prostate cancer—a hot topic among us boys. I kid my friends: We used to talk about girls and cars, now it's prostates and diverticulitis.

I take a nap this afternoon, the first one I've taken since I found out that I had prostate cancer. I feel slightly depressed. Or is it simply a letdown after everything I've been through, now that it's over?

No letdown in urinary urgency, though. That "runs on" unabated.

Funny. The weather's gorgeous here, cold at home, but I've already begun thinking how nice it will be to go home. I miss the dogs.

Friday March 2

Day 16. The "letdown" is actually a virus, which is probably why I took the nap.

I was wiped out last evening and had to lie down on the couch. I could tell I was definitely coming down with something. Could my immune system have been compromised by the radiation?

Because lymphoid tissue controls the immune system, radiation can suppress the immune system if lymphoid tissue is irradiated. But radiation of the prostate gland should cause minimal immune system suppression because little lymphoid tissue is irradiated.

I instant-message with Carol in California. "Two male friends here have prostate cancer and are trying to decide what to do," she says. "Why did you choose radiation?"

I tell her. She is very interested. "Prostate cancer's a hot topic out here," she says.

Saturday March 3

Day 17. Coughing from the chest, a viral bronchitis, sapping my energy and appetite. I'm quite sure it's not related to radiation.

I'm taking plenty of fluids, and because of my continuing urinary urgency I don't want to get too far from the bathroom.

Sunday March 4

Day 18. I instant-message again with Carol in California. "Our two friends have decided on surgery," she says. "They just want the cancer out."

Who can blame them? I think. But do they know all the possible complications? Some men have their minds made up and just want the cancer out of their bodies.

"Men we know who've had the surgery had complications but were back to normal after 18 months," says Carol.

"That's not true of everyone with complications," I say. "And there can be difficulties with men reporting complications like incontinence and impotence."

"That's probably true," she says. "Guys might have trouble admitting to embarrassing problems."

Monday March 5

Day 19. No apparent complications related to the radiation.

I talk about prostate cancer with Allen, a retired Ear, Nose, and Throat doctor. "Most of the boys," he says, "are getting surgery."

What Do Tomatoes, Vitamin E, and Oily Fish Have in Common?

Tomatoes, vitamin E, and oily fish are more than just ingredients for a healthy chowder. They may all have the ability to fight prostate cancer.

Tomatoes

Several studies have linked tomatoes with a reduction in prostate cancer, and the agent most likely responsible for this is lycopene, the red pigment that gives tomatoes and tomato sauces their color. Lycopene is a potent antioxidant, and antioxidants are thought to help fight cancer by protecting cells from damage.

Processed, cooked, or concentrated tomatoes appear to be more beneficial than raw tomatoes because cooking breaks down the cell walls of the tomatoes, releasing more lycopene. In fact, five times the amount of lycopene is absorbed by the body from tomato sauce than from an equivalent quantity of raw tomatoes. In addition, tomatoes cooked in oil seem more easily absorbed by the body, probably because lycopene is fat-soluble.

Lycopene can also be found in such fruits as watermelon and pink grapefruit. It may not be stored in the body for long and therefore should be replenished at least twice a week.

Lycopene appears effective not only in preventing prostate cancer but in retarding it as well. In one Harvard study, men who ate more tomato sauce had a significantly lower risk of developing prostate cancer. Of men with prostate cancer, those eating more tomato sauce were less likely to experience metastasis, or spread, of their disease.

In another study from the University of Illinois at Chicago, prostate cancer patients were fed one tomato-based pasta dish per day for three weeks, each entrée (stuffed shells, penne pasta, sausage lasagna, and baked rigatoni) containing 3/4 of a cup of tomato sauce. Over the three-week period, the amount of lycopene in the participants' blood and prostate tissue increased, while damage due to oxidation, which has been linked to cancer, decreased. The patients' PSA levels also dropped, suggesting that the number of cancer cells might have diminished.

Vitamin E
A study in Finland has found that participants who took three times the recommended daily allowance of vitamin E had 32 percent fewer cases of prostate cancer and 41 percent fewer deaths from prostate cancer than those who did not take vitamin E supplements. It is possible that vitamin E may prevent relatively benign cancer cells from progressing to a more malignant stage. However, a small number of men in the study who took vitamin E developed hemorrhagic strokes. This possible side effect of vitamin E needs careful study before vitamin E supplements can be recommended for prostate health.

Oily Fish
A report from Sweden concludes that men who never eat fish have two to three times the risk of prostate cancer than those eating moderate or large amounts of fish. The investigators point out that only oily fish, such as mackerel, salmon, sardines, and herring—all of which contain high amounts of omega-3 fatty acids—provide this benefit.

New Zealand researchers found a clear connection between high levels of fish oil in the blood and a reduced incidence of prostate cancer. They divided the men studied into 4 equal groups, depending on the level of fish oil in their blood. The men in the group with the highest levels of fish oil in their blood had a 40 percent lower rate of prostate cancer than the men with the least amount of fish oil.

Tuesday March 6

Day 20. My laptop won't turn on this morning, which scares the hell out of me, because I depend on it—I mean depend on it—to write. Trevor and Sarah give me a ride to the computer store. On the way we discuss—what else?—prostate-related issues, including urgency. They understand what I'm talking about. It sounds as if Trevor has benign prostatic hyperplasia. Prostates, prostates everywhere.

Wednesday March 7

Day 21. We bump into Fred, one of the guys I play tennis with, at a bar tonight, and like a perfect bore I begin to enumerate the maladies I've suffered in the recent past. He stops me at prostate cancer.

"How did you treat it?" he asks.

"Radiation," I say. "Finished just before we came down here."

"I had prostate cancer, too," he says. "I went to the university hospital where they do nerve-sparing surgery. My urologist was a cold fish. We discussed surgery, but the complications were never fully spelled out. 'You might have some sexual dysfunction,' he said, 'but you'll be all right.' That's bullshit. I had surgery and haven't had an erection since, and never will. I'm also incontinent. I dribble a little playing tennis. Wearing a catheter for weeks was the worst part of the surgery. I hated it."

He looks at me. "What about complications from radiation? Aren't they about the same as from surgery?"

(I would later find out that Fred is a financial analyst, a smart guy. But he wasn't knowledgeable about the treatment of his own prostate cancer.)

"No," I say, and start telling him the differences.

He puts up a hand to stop me. "Never mind." He isn't interested in talking about it. He's chosen his mode of treatment, and though it hasn't worked out ideally, he has no choice but to live with it.

Fred is 62, like me. "I have a very understanding wife," he says. "I've tried injections to get an erection, but the spontaneity is gone. It's frustrating."

He orders another drink. "I get follow-up questionnaires from the hospital about every six months. They ask how I'm doing. I don't answer. What man wants to admit he can't get it up? My new urologist is a real sweet guy, which really helps, but the surgeon was a cold fish."

Why does someone like this, who is so clearly dissatisfied with his medical care, not voice his dissatisfactions to his surgeon or to the institution where he had his surgery? I think because Fred would have to disclose things that are humiliating to him and he doesn't want to do that.

In her last instant-message, Carol remarked that "guys might have trouble admitting to embarrassing problems." Fred obviously does.

Given the reluctance of men to discuss their sexual problems, can we trust follow-up studies on prostate cancer therapy? The investigators might not be getting straight answers or the whole story. Fred won't respond to the questionnaires. He has complications that won't be included in the statistics of the hospital where he had his surgery.

Thursday March 8

Day 22. I have a recurring dream about performing orthopedic surgery. Last night I had one that seemed to go on and on. I was detoured, delayed, couldn't get to the surgical suite to operate on a young woman already under anesthesia. When I finally did arrive, I struggled to prep myself for the operation. I woke up with a feeling of gloom and doom.

I'm squirming, wriggling out the other end of a week's viral infestation of my body.

I bump into Fred, the financial analyst, and his wife, Karen. She fears that urologists don't always lay out all the facts before doing prostate cancer surgery.

"Perhaps," I say, "he told you more than you think, and in the anxiety of the moment you didn't absorb it."

She nods. "Perhaps."

"I'm convinced that urologists have no doubt that surgery is the best treatment for prostate cancer," I say. "It's been the gold standard for years. I also think they believe they present complications pre-operatively in a fair and clear manner. Mine did."

"Ours didn't," says Karen.

"But let me tell you something," I say. "I know an orthopedist who used to give a comprehensive list of possible complications to his patients before total joint replacement. What did it do? Scared them off. Once they learned the bad things that can happen—even if they rarely do—they decided against surgery, even though they needed it. So what did the orthopedist do? Stopped giving out the list, stopped explaining all the potential complications. He didn't want to deprive his patients of a surgery he knew that they needed. He still informed them of complications, but not as extensively as before. Might that help explain something about urologists? Convinced that for prostate cancer surgery is the best option, they may not want to deprive the patient of having it."

Monday March 12

Day 26. Bowel irritation is basically gone, urinary urgency better, but still some hesitancy on starting urination, and some urethral irritation—not burning, just a sensation of urine passing through it.

Tuesday March 13

Day 27. No blood in my stools for days. I have been eating a lot of fiber, from cauliflower, broccoli, carrots, and tomatoes. I've been buying so many veggies I even know how to spell them correctly now.

I'm feeling good for perhaps the first time since my knee surgery last July. Let's see ... surgery, bleeding into the joint afterwards, physical therapy, prostate biopsy, dental work, colonoscopy, radiation, viral bronchitis—I'm probably missing a few things. It's hell growing old.

Wednesday March 14

Day 28. Our friend Greg phones. "Larry, a guy I used to work with," he says, "has a PSA around 6, no biopsy done. You've tried making sense of this subject for other people."

"I've tried making sense of it for myself," I say.

"Do you mind if he calls you for information or advice? He lives in Los Angeles."

"Not at all, have him call."

Thursday March 15

Day 29. Blood in stool for the first time in quite a while.

Friday March 16

Day 30. I have a sensation in the urethra that I think is related to the radiation. It's not uncomfortable, just there. Pretty amazing that I got through all the radiation with so few side effects. If the radiation has killed the cancer cells as it was supposed to, what an excellent form of treatment! Think of the alternatives. I might be at home struggling with surgical complications rather than playing tennis in Florida.

Saturday March 17

Day 31. Hubert, a 60-year-old stock broker from Pennsylvania, underwent a radical prostatectomy 10 months ago. He is still having problems.

"My Gleason score was 5. I knew about radiation, but I just wanted to get the cancer out, so I chose surgery."

I get the feeling that he doesn't quite understand the difference between seeds and external beam radiation. To him it is all just radiation.

Complementary and Alternative Treatments for Prostate Cancer

I strongly recommend conventional medical methods (surgery, radiation, and cryotherapy) as primary treatments for prostate cancer. But many men may justifiably wish to integrate alternative approaches into their medical care.

Some common complementary, or alternative, therapies include herbs, nutritional supplements, acupuncture, naturopathy, massage and physical therapy, reflexology, traditional Chinese medicine, spiritual support, mind-body medicine (or psychoneuro-immunology), and image enhancement.

Many herbal remedies are currently being marketed for prostate health, but the American Cancer Society warns that, because herbs are considered dietary supplements and not drugs, they are not strictly tested and regulated by the FDA. According to the American Cancer Society, "the only dietary supplement to show some benefit against prostate cancer in well-conducted scientific studies, known as PC-SPES, was pulled off the market in 2002 when it was discovered to be contaminated with prescription drugs."

Two substances frequently mentioned in the context of prostate cancer treatment are selenium and saw palmetto. Selenium is an essential mineral found in many foods. Several recent studies show that selenium lowers the risk of prostate cancer. A large study sponsored by the National Cancer Institute is currently underway to evaluate whether selenium and vitamin E can help prevent prostate cancer. However, the National Academy of Science cautions that too much selenium can cause undesirable side effects.

While effective for treating benign prostatic hyperplasia (enlargement of the prostate), saw palmetto, a widely available herb, has not been shown to be effective against prostate cancer. Furthermore, saw palmetto can lower the PSA level and potentially shroud an existing prostate cancer. Therefore, any use of saw palmetto must be supervised by a physician.

A study at the University of Virginia found that 43 percent of prostate cancer patients use at least one alternative or complementary treatment in addition to their conventional treatment. The complementary treatments most frequently used were vitamins, herbal medicines, and prayer and other spiritual practices. Younger patients and those with high Gleason scores were more likely to use alternative remedies.

Perhaps the most troubling caveat from this study was that 72 percent of patients using alternative methods do not tell their doctors what they are doing. While complementary methods can be helpful, they can also do harm if they interfere with the primary method of treatment. It is imperative that you tell your physician about any complementary or alternative medicines or treatments that you are using to deal with your prostate cancer.

"Since surgery," he says, "my energy level's been down. I can't play tennis and golf on the same day the way I used to. I get tired in the third set in tennis. Never used to do that.

"After surgery I got a bladder infection, then a urethral stricture and couldn't pass my urine. They stretched the stricture two or three times, but then said they couldn't do that anymore. So when I go home from here I'm scheduled for a cutting of the narrowed area."

This worries me. What do they do if this additional surgery doesn't work?

"I have no problem with impotence," he says, but then he describes his sexual performance. "Sometimes I get an erection, sometimes I don't, whereas I used to get one just looking at something. I sometimes take Viagra, and it's getting better."

He treats all this as though it were routine, to be expected. "Patients are back to normal 18 months after surgery," he says.

Carol has said the same thing. I wonder where this claim comes from?

"I'll be fine," says Hubert.

"Did you learn what complications could occur before you had your surgery?" I ask.

Hubert's a nice guy. "The surgeon's a busy man," he says, "and didn't explain them all." He shrugs his shoulders. "That's the way it goes."

He's stuck with these problems. He minimizes them. but who can blame him? Life goes on.

Learning you have cancer alarms and confuses you. Dr. Bruce told me that when a patient learns he has cancer, he hears only a small portion of what's discussed after that—treatment options, outcomes of therapy, side effects, complications. While trying to decide on a course of action, a man's judgment is often cloudy at best.

Both Hubert, a successful broker, and Fred, a successful financial analyst, had difficulties understanding what they were getting into. If these savvy, experienced men weren't fully informed when they made their decisions, how many other men must be equally uninformed?

No one can fault Hubert for wanting the cancer removed. We all do when we're told we have cancer. I did. My wife did. But then we sat down and found out that there are other ways to treat the cancer.

Monday March 19

Day 33. There is blood in my stool. I just need to eat more veggies. I'm sure it's not serious.

We don't have veggies and aren't about to go shopping on our bikes in the rain, so I take a fiber supplement this afternoon. Dr. Kennedy recommended it, and I'll see how it goes.

Wednesday March 21

Day 35. A friend's here from Washington, D.C. "Four of my buddies have prostate cancer," he says. "Two had surgery, two had seeds. The two with surgery are completely impotent."

Thursday March 22

Day 36. Urethral irritation improving; still some urgency.

Friday March 23

Day 37. Took a bus to go shopping. But having taken the fiber supplement and still dealing with urinary urgency, I am a bit uneasy about getting too far from a bathroom.

We enjoy a great lunch. I don't drink much water, and am I glad I don't. I urinate at the restaurant and again at a department store, then wait over an hour for the bus to take us home. It never comes. Finally we take a taxi.

Monday March 26

Day 40. Phone message from Greg's friend Larry in Los Angeles. He'll call tomorrow to discuss his prostate problems.

Tuesday March 27

Day 41. Larry calls again. "Thanks for talking to me. I'm an old friend of Greg, who called you about me. My PSA went from 3.7 to 5.5."

"That doesn't necessarily mean you have cancer," I say.

"Really? I thought it did."

I tell him about other factors that can elevate PSA.

"I'm glad to hear that," he says. "My biopsy is in a couple of weeks."

I tell him why I chose external beam radiation and why urologists are inclined to recommend surgery.

Friday March 30

Day 44. Warming up for tennis, my doubles partner says to me, "I'm coming off back surgery, and I don't feel I can move around too freely."

"Not to worry," I say. "I'm getting over knee surgery and can't move real well myself."

I call across the net to one of our opponents—Reed, a retired Army officer. I tell him we might not be able to run down every ball, and why.

He ambles toward the net grinning from ear to ear. "That's fine, I've got a total hip replacement."

As Tom, our fourth, strolls onto the court, I fill him in on our physical limitations.

"No problem," he says. "I've had a quadruple heart bypass."

This is the way it is with us old farts nowadays. But we have a good game anyway.

Saturday March 31

Day 45. My urinary urgency continues to improve. I think I'm coming out of this thing.

Wednesday April 11

Day 56. The weather beautiful, but we go home on Friday. We're ready to see the dogs. Sleeping in our own bed will be okay, too.

Friday April 13

Day 58. Friday the thirteenth, Good Friday, and our travel day.

Saturday April 14

Day 59. It's nice being home again. My urethral symptoms are better, and my urinary urgency is much better.

Monday April 16

Day 61. I have to schedule a follow-up PSA. I am a little scared thinking about it. What do we do if it's 7, or 27? Start looking for cancer all over again?

I phone Dr. Bruce. "How are you doing?" he asks.

"No blood in stools lately," I say, "and the urinary symptoms are better."

"Fine, schedule a follow-up visit and a PSA."

Wednesday April 18.

Day 63. I go to the hospital and have blood drawn for the PSA test. While waiting in an examining room for Dr. Bruce, I chat with one of the oncology nurses.

"I know a man who received his diagnosis of prostate cancer from the urologist by telephone at 10:00 on a Friday night, and had to wait the weekend for more information," she says.

"Must've been a long weekend," I say. "I got my diagnosis at 5:00. But it was on a Monday."

Emerging Technologies for Treating Prostate Cancer

Intensity Modulated Radiation Therapy
Intensity Modulated Radiation Therapy (IMRT) is the state of the art for delivering external beam radiation. IMRT breaks radiation into tiny packets of radiation beams, allowing for greater accuracy in striking a targeted area than older radiation techniques. IMRT can deliver a higher radiation dose to cancerous tumors and hit more specific areas within a tumor, while giving a lower dose to surrounding tissues, thereby decreasing treatment toxicity. While IMRT can be used to treat some types of previously radiated tumors, it cannot be used to re-radiate a prostate cancer tumor.

Proton Beam Radiation
Another new form of radiation is proton beam radiation, in which the radiation beams are made up of microscopic particles called protons. An advantage of this therapy is that the particles cause little damage going through normal healthy tissue, such as skin, and can be concentrated to kill cancer cells at a specified location. Although proton beam radiation is being used for prostate cancer, it is not widely available because the particles must be created in large cyclotrons, which few institutions have access to.

Laparoscopic and Robotic-Laparoscopic Prostatectomy
Instead of a single large abdominal incision, laparoscopic radical prostatectomy requires only a few small 1/4- to 1/2-inch abdominal incisions. This minimally invasive surgery is done with a miniaturized camera and extremely small instruments. The advantages of laparoscopic prostatectomy over traditional open prostatectomy include less blood loss, quicker removal of the catheter, and faster recovery. Whether there is less risk of complications such as incontinence and impotence is not yet clear.

Some medical centers are now performing laparoscopic prostatectomies with the aid of sophisticated robotics. In a robotically assisted laparoscopic prostatectomy, the surgeon sits at a console in front of a wide projection screen manipulating robotic arms and tiny instruments inside the abdomen. The advantages of this technology are greater precision of control, improved view of anatomical structures, and the potential for reducing the risks of side effects, including impotence and incontinence.

Immunotherapy and Gene Therapy
In the future, immunotherapy and gene therapy may well become the treatments of choice for prostate cancer. Unlike current treatments that damage healthy cells along with the cancerous ones, immunotherapy and gene therapy attack only the cancerous cells, whether localized in the prostate gland or spread to other parts of the body. At least this is the theory behind the research in this area. But research is moving slowly. Because human beings are the only species commonly afflicted with prostate cancer, there are no really good animal models for research.

The goal of immunotherapy is to develop a vaccine that would cause the body's natural immune system to attack prostate cancer cells as if they were foreign intruders. The difficulty is finding antigens specific to the prostate cancer cell. But if an antibody carrying a toxic agent could be made to attach itself to a prostate cancer cell, it could theoretically kill that cell while leaving all other cells in the body intact.

There are two promising avenues of research in gene therapy. Because many cancers have mutated genes that cause their cells to grow and behave wildly, researchers are hopeful they may be able either to introduce a factor into a cancer cell which affects only the mutated gene or to replace a malfunctioning gene with a normal gene. But different patients develop different mutations, and getting normal genes into every cell of an organ remains a major challenge. At this time, virtually all immunotherapy and gene therapy for prostate cancer is experimental.

"Dr. Bruce is getting pressure from urologists who send him patients for consultation and then don't get them back when they choose radiation over surgery. Dr. Bruce is a good man and a great physician. You know, I started in radiation oncology 10 years ago. Nowadays we see a lot less complications than we did then."

"Better targeting of the intended area."

She talks about physicians who contract cancer. "I knew a neurosurgeon who developed a severe brain tumor, and it changed his practice and his partners'. They became much more sympathetic toward their patients. But seven or eight years later, they went back to their old ways."

She once asked her husband whether he would be willing to inject his penis before sex. "No way," he replied. She then asked him whether he would do if it was the only way he could ever have sex again. "I'd learn," he said.

"A prostate cancer support group began at this hospital 10 years ago and became defunct a year ago," she says. "It was a very active group, with speakers and discussions. I don't know why it went under."

"Once I'm beyond treatment and feeling well," I say, "the last thing I'll want to do is come back and relive the treatments, complications, side effects people go through. Maybe that's why it ended."

"But patients coming into this situation need to talk to people like you. When the diagnosis comes, it's a shock."

"Certainly was to me."

"The patient hears how treatment will be from a doctor or nurse, but it's not the same as from a person who's been through it."

Dr. Bruce arrives and examines my prostate. "It's still enlarged, but not very much and I found no nodules. How have you been doing?"

"No urinating at night," I say. "Urinary urgency and frequency seem pretty much at pre-radiation levels. No blood in stools for a month. No sexual dysfunction. I'm feeling good."

"If your PSA is up, we'll get another one in a month or two, but no tests to look for a spread of your cancer before then. I'll call you tomorrow with today's test result."

Thursday April 19

Day 64. At 7:45 a.m. the telephone rings. I answer in the pantry next to the kitchen. "Your PSA is 1.18," says Dr. Bruce, "a very good, low number, and I would expect it to continue going down."

"I'm happy to hear that," I say.

"Come back in three months for another PSA and exam."

Fantastic, I think, hanging up. My last PSA, drawn right after my first radiation treatment, was 6.28. Now I know for sure that there really was something coming out of that big noisy machine.

I call the news excitedly up the stairs to Ilka. "Great!" she says.

I phone my brother Jack, and he is happy. "I treated lots of testicular tumors," he says. "That's a cancer with a good serum marker, a blood test like the PSA for prostate cancer. The tests were drawn every three months. If the result was good, the patient and his family were relieved for the next six weeks. But their anxiety would mount for the six weeks after that, the test looming ever closer. It's a roller coaster ride, and you can expect some of that."

"I'm sure," I say. "But I feel good now."

His wife gets on the phone. "Doing all the research you did before selecting a treatment was so smart."

At this point, I think so too.

I call my friend Todd at work with the good news. I phone our son David and my cousin Ellen and my friend Mark, but they aren't answering. (How can this be?) I call Greg, and Kelly is there, and I tell her. She suggests I call Don, and he isn't home. (How dare he be out when I have such exciting news to share!) I phone Delores, and she isn't there. What's going on? I leave messages for David and Ellen. But—no one to tell?

Sunday April 22

Day 67. Gloomy, rainy, and cold outside. But inside? Bowel and bladder are functioning flawlessly.

Tuesday April 24

Day 69. Bright, sunny day. Baseball cap in place.

Tonight a long program about prostate cancer produced by the Memorial Sloan Kettering Cancer Center airs on the Discovery Channel. Ilka summons me to watch.

"It's important," she says, "that we be up on everything about prostate cancer."

She's right. The program is about three men taking a vaccine for prostate cancer as a last resort and enjoying encouraging results. I have to hope that should I ever get to a point of last resort, treatments will have improved dramatically from where they are now. But my real hope is that I never get to the point of last resort.

Friday April 27

Day 72. A beautiful spring day. No blood in my stool; my urinary urgency is down. This makes the day even more beautiful. It seems that Dr. Bruce did a good job aiming those rays.

I pick up my car from the repair shop, turn the corner onto our street, and stop. Doug comes down from his driveway. "How's your health?" he asks.

"Pretty good," I say. "My latest PSA was down."

When you have cancer, people don't forget.

Saturday April 28

Day 73. When I tell people my recent PSA was 1.18, they cheerfully assume the disease has been knocked out. I hope they're right. But I know it's possible they're not.

Monday April 30

Day 75. I have a long phone conversation with Larry from California. "A week ago," he says, "the urologist called and said I have prostate cancer. The biopsy showed it in 2 of the 8 specimens taken. My Gleason score is 7, and he recommended surgery. He was frank about the chance of impotence, saying it was a coin flip. He said incontinence occurs in about 5 percent of surgery patients. I'll see a radiation oncologist on Wednesday."

"You might even want a third opinion," I say. I tell him about the BAT system. "You might consider coming back here if you choose external beam radiation."

"Seeding was initiated in Seattle. I think I'll go there if I choose seeds."

We talk about some of the information I've researched.

"E-mail me addresses for the web sites that were most helpful," he says.

Poor Larry's going through the same thing I went through several months ago. I know what he feels like.

"How's your wife doing?" I ask.

"She alternates between depression and being semi-okay."

Tuesday May 1

Day 76. I think again about Larry this morning, and the unenviable position he's in—that I *was* in—trying to make a decision—a position many, many men find themselves in every day.

Thursday May 3

Day 78. I speak again with Larry. "I saw a radiation oncologist yesterday," he says. "He does both 3D-CRT and temporary seeds. I mentioned to the doctor that temporary seeds apparently hadn't worked for Andy Grove of Intel. He said he knew the physician who did that procedure, and would call him and find out what happened."

Larry chuckles. "After talking to the surgeon, I thought I'd have surgery, just cut the sucker out. After reading a book on seeds, I thought that would be the way to go. After seeing the radiation oncologist, I thought I should do external beam. It seems whoever I talk to last will be the one I choose."

"It's hard making a decision," I say. I tell him about the nuisance of having your bladder full for 3D-CRT and my experience the first time there.

"I read that you have to drink three or four cups of water beforehand," he says. "That's a lot of water."

Tell me about it.

He's going on vacation for a week. "I'm taking stuff about prostate cancer to read. I'll try to decide what to do in the next two weeks."

Saturday May 5

Day 80. I send Larry an e-mail with websites I've bookmarked on my browser while researching prostate cancer. Quite a few no longer exist—the evanescence of information on the Internet.

Monday May 7

Day 82. Bright and sunny. Sure am happy when I think about my PSA. I feel I did the right thing in choosing radiation.

Saturday May 12

Day 87. "What's happening with your prostate cancer?" our next-door neighbor asks me.

"Seems under control," I say. "I should say I hope it's under control."

Monday May 14

Day 89. If there's less ejaculate after prostate radiation, would it be more difficult to impregnate a woman? Is fertility compromised?

Tuesday May 15

Day 90. Mary, Don's wife, calls. "Don finished radiation four weeks ago," she says, "and had almost no side effects, just a little diarrhea treated with an over-

> Radiation *can* affect fertility. If you are a younger man wishing to father children, you should consider banking your sperm before you undergo radiation therapy.

the-counter anti-diarrheal. But a relative of mine went through prostate surgery a few weeks ago and has just been floored by it— incontinent and very unhappy about the whole thing being as extreme as it was."

"Sorry to her about your relative, but it's good news about Don," I say. "I have good news, too. My recent PSA was 1.18."

"That's wonderful. Don and I are very happy we talked with you. Only then did we realize what can happen with surgery. Our urologist made it seem so minor."

Thursday May 17

Day 92. Mary calls again. "Don's very pleased with your latest PSA. He'll have one drawn soon and ... we're concerned about it."

"My brother was a pediatric oncologist," I say. "He treated testicular cancer patients who had a blood test similar to the PSA, drawn every three months. If the result was good, they had six weeks of relief, then six weeks of anxiety—a real up and down ride."

"I'm afraid we're in for that, too."

Friday May 18

Day 93. I speak with Larry in Los Angeles. "I got your websites," he says. "I've put all the data I collected on a spreadsheet. Man, have I got information up the kazoo, but I'll make a decision in a couple of weeks. Tell me again about radiation's effects."

I tell him about my urinary and rectal urgency.

"That's not bad," he says. "I thought by 'rectal urgency' you meant if you weren't near a toilet you'd crap in your pants."

"It wasn't quite that way. I did have four or five bowel movements a day and more urgency to urinate than usual, but that's all gone now."

Saturday May 19

Day 94. Dinner, then a concert. I am very familiar with the route, having taken it for each of my 42 radiation treatments. I don't mention it to the others. I just know the road.

Monday May 21

Day 96. At a reception, my ears prick up when I overhear a man say something in conversation with another person: "I'm on Lupron, a hormone which shuts down the male hormone testosterone."

I turn to him. "Do you have prostate cancer?"

Looking surprised, he replies, "I do, and take Lupron and another drug for it."

"I have prostate cancer, too," I say, and we begin an extended conversation. He talks freely about his disease. He seems healthy and has a keen mind. I don't know his age, but would guess he's at least 80.

"My Gleason score was 6," he says. "I saw several physicians before choosing my treatment. The first surgeon I saw was on his way out the door when he stopped and turned to me. 'Give two or three pints of blood,' he said, 'because we tend to lose quite a bit during surgery.' Then he turned again and just kept on walking. I never went back to him. Would you?"

"I don't think so."

"I saw another surgeon, went to the Mayo Clinic, and finally saw a physician in Sarasota, Florida, who puts in seeds. I had him do it, and a couple of years later my PSA shot up to 7 or 8. They put me on hormones, and I'm still on them, and not very happy about it. My breasts are bigger than my wife's." He chuckles. "My PSA's down, and that's fine, but so's everything else."

He eyes me. "Know anything about cryosurgery?"

"Not much, only that they freeze tissue, and one doctor told me it might be a viable alternative for treating prostate cancer in the near future."

He looks away. "Let me tell you something strange. This is a man's disease, yet the doctors I saw all men seemed entirely unconcerned about it. I don't know why, but I don't like it."

Tuesday May 29

Day 104. I speak with Larry. "Still trying to make a decision," he says. "I'm going to a medical oncologist in a couple of weeks who asked me to get a second opinion on my biopsy because the Gleason score is critical to the treatment you choose. If the score's 7, the treatment is radiation. If it's 6, the treatment is surgery. My pathology slides are being sent to UCLA and Stanford. We'll see what happens."

Friday June 1

Day 107. An e-mail from Larry contains an article by a radiation oncologist in Michigan. It says that 40 percent of prostate cancer treatment in this country is through external beam radiation and the results from radiation therapy are as good as or better than radical prostatectomy.

According the article, the American Urologic Association Prostate Cancer Guideline Panel has analyzed all available information on radiation and surgery, and declared that there is "no clear-cut evidence for the superiority of any one treatment."

The article goes on to say that 40 to 56 percent of patients treated with external beam radiation for all stages of prostate cancer have a PSA that is stable after 5 years. A patient with early stage disease treated with radiation has an 80 to 90 percent chance of having a stable PSA at 5 years, which is the same as the best surgical reports.

The article describes the possible side effects from radiation, including proctitis and cystitis. Larry asks in his e-mail what these are. I write back that proctitis is inflammation of the rectum and cystitis is inflammation of the bladder.

One long-term effect of external beam radiation, according to the article, is impotence, occurring in about half the patients. That's interesting, because it doesn't jibe with the 1999 study from Fox Chase Cancer Center in Philadelphia, a study I discussed with Dr. Bruce. The Philadelphia study showed excellent post-3D-CRT sexual function in men with prostate cancer who were 65 years old or younger. I suspect the finding in Larry's article is related to older, less accurate radiation techniques.

Sunday June 3

Day 109. On the way to brunch I tell my wife that I have a pain in my right buttock. "It started with what I thought was a hamstring pull in Florida. It's evolved into a pain in the butt (quite literally), with some vague radiation down the back of my upper thigh. I also have numbness in the right heel and little toe. I've been waiting for it all to go away. It hasn't."

Monday June 4

Day 110. I doubt the buttock pain has anything to do with my prostate cancer. Five days after getting home from Florida my PSA was 1.18, and it would probably have been higher had the cancer spread to bone. But I'll call Dr. Ted Morton, an orthopedist, and get it checked out. Ilka agrees with this idea. The pain might be from the sciatic nerve or a ruptured disc.

Wednesday June 6

Day 112. Don calls. He's doing well and has a post-radiation PSA of 3. Good for him.

Thursday June 7

Day 113. I see Dr. Morton, and the pain is fairly severe as he examines me. He takes X-rays of my pelvis and right hip. They appear normal.

"I don't think the pain's coming from your back or sciatic nerve," he says. "But because you underwent prostate radiation, I'd like to get MRI scans of your right hip and pelvis. Radiation can cause avascular necrosis of the femoral head. That might be causing your pain."

This, I think as I leave, would not be good. In fact, it would be very bad.

"Avascular necrosis of the femoral head" simply means that the ball portion of the ball and socket in the hip joint is dead. In such cases, the ball at the end of the femur, or large leg bone, collapses, and major hip surgery, usually a total hip replacement, is required to fix it.

As soon as I get home I call Dr. Bruce. "I'm not at all concerned about your having that," he says. "Was the doctor a young guy or older?"

"On the older side," I say.

"In the old days the bone did get significant radiation, but with modern techniques and high energy radiation the bone gets so little that I'm not worried about it."

"That makes me feel better."

Tuesday June 12

Day 118. I have a long phone conversation with Larry. He has been alarmed by an article about cryotherapy and has sent me a copy of it in an e-mail.

The article appears to be a press release from a brokerage house. It advises investors to purchase stock in a company producing an array of cryotherapy equipment. The article asserts that the company stands to gain the entire prostate cancer radiation market within the next 12 to 24 months. The assertion is based on several claims, including the claim that urologists are beginning to believe that radiation is carcinogenic, causing cancer in healthy cells; that the impotency rate for external beam radiation patients is 40 percent; and that 30,000 brachytherapy patients per year will turn to cryotherapy as failure rates for brachytherapy increase dramatically.

"I was upset after reading this," says Larry, "because I've basically decided on external beam radiation."

"This article borders on being unethical in stating that cryosurgery will totally take over radiation treatment in the next one to two years," I say. "Furthermore, while older radiation therapies did have impotency rates of 50 percent or more, the rates appear to be much lower when 3D-CRT is used. And while radiation therapy is carcinogenic, this is not an issue for most prostate cancer patients because of their age. Radiation-induced cancer is only a concern for younger people—say, children or breast cancer patients in their 40s. And as for the article's suggestion that seed patients might be showing tumor recurrence in large numbers, that's simply not the case."

Larry seems to settle down as we talk.

"The article points out that a huge problem with cryosurgery is impotence—80 percent," he says. "I've talked to three men who had prostate surgery. Two are impotent, but they might have had larger, more complicated surgeries than usual. The third guy's function didn't come back until months afterwards. Well, I'm taking a long time making a decision, aren't I? A couple of months so far."

"You have to be comfortable with it," I say.

"My family doctor's been bugging me. 'All your choices are good,' he says. 'Just get going.'"

"You'll have doubts along the way—after reaching a decision, during treatment, even after it's over. I've had all the above. You can only hope the chosen treatment does its job, and the tumor doesn't return in any way, shape, or form."

After we hang up, I begin thinking about my MRI exams scheduled for tonight. I phone my son David, who's a neuroradiology fellow in San Francisco, where they do tons of MRIs.

"What's it like for the patient?" I ask. "You know I'm claustrophobic."

"Take a CD with you," he says, "and—at least where I work—they'll play it for you while your scan's being done."

I pick a CD and take a tranquilizer before Ilka drives me to the imaging facility.

I'm glad I took the tranquilizer. Lying on my back, I am pushed into a fairly constrictive tube, but I am happy to see that the other end is open. The technicians play my CD, but the sound quality is poor and the machine, during its runs, clunks, bangs, and buzzes so loudly it is hard to hear anything else. I have a moment's nervousness, but then fall into a light sleep.

The session takes 40 minutes and is doubtless longer than usual because two separate exams have to be done: the hip and pelvis.

"Good job," says a male technician. "You held really still. We got good pictures."

I'll get a report tomorrow when I see Dr. Nathan, my old friend and family doctor.

Wednesday June 13

Day 119. Dr. Nathan holds a report of the scans. "What do you want first," he asks, "the good news or the bad news?"

"The bad news," I say.

"The pain's coming from a partial tear of the common hamstring tendon off the pelvic bone. It's a hamstring tear, way up high. It'll take time to heal, but it will heal."

"The good news?"

"The pain's not coming from a spread of your cancer, the sciatic nerve, or a dead femoral head. We'll get you started in physical therapy."

Wednesday June 20

I can't remember the last time I got up during the night to urinate, and my urinary urgency is better. No blood in my stools for a couple of months.

Thursday June 28

A reminder on my calendar to call Dr. Bruce's office for an appointment in a couple of weeks, which makes me a little nervous. I don't know what my PSA will be. Can't we just leave well enough alone? I'm feeling fine, except for the hamstring, which is slowly mending.

Friday June 29

I speak with Larry. "My Gleason score is 7," he says. "This means there's a 60 percent chance the cancer's gone beyond the capsule, the prostate's lining. I will need more than just external beam radiation. I'm considering getting the seeds in Seattle, or 3D-CRT at UCLA with hormones before and during the radiation.

"I'm seeing Dr. Mark Scholz, a medical oncologist treating prostate cancer only. He gave me nomographs, charts dealing with numerical relationships, success rates for surgery and external beam radiation using various PSA values and Gleason scores. In working them out, it's assumed you go to the best places for treatment—a top surgeon for prostatectomy, the Cleveland Clinic for external beam, and Seattle for seeds.

"I worked them out using my PSA and Gleason and found the cure rate for me from surgery would be 86 percent, and from external beam 89 percent. I don't have a nomograph for seeds, but I think the percentage would be similar to external beam, maybe higher, because you can get a higher dose inside the gland."

So Larry's still thinking hard.

Sunday July 1

With this hamstring injury, I'm unable to get exercise in my usual ways. Going stir crazy, I borrow a bike from our neighbor across the street. I find that I can peddle without pain and end up going all the way around the lake. Last summer I biked around the lake once and was surprised by how uncomfortable the seat was and how jarring the bike path was. Today I revel in every bump and the seat feels fine.

As one guy passes me (all the bikers do), I almost turn to him and say, "Look at me. I'm biking!"

Monday July 9

I call Dr. Bruce's office. In two days I go in for a PSA. Some anxiety about it, thinking about that evening after it's drawn, waiting for the phone call the next day.

I would like to continue biking for exercise, but I have definite concerns about it. Dr. Fitzgerald, my urologist, once mentioned to me that the PSA level can go up from riding a bike.

With a PSA test coming up in a few days, the last thing I want is bump up my PSA on a bicycle seat.

I've heard of bike saddles that are split down the middle to keep pressure off vulnerable anatomical structures, including the prostate. I have no idea how common these seats are, or how to find one.

It turns out it isn't hard at all. I search the Internet for local bicycle shops and find one nearby. Lo and behold, the shop sells divided seats. I go there right away. The shop carries two models, one for males and one for females, the one for females having a wider gap.

"I want to protect my prostate," I tell the young salesman.

"Take the female model," he says.

"It's for girls."

He gives me a hard look. "If I wanted to protect my prostate, I wouldn't let that worry me."

I purchase a beautiful white bike with 21 gears made in China— and the female seat.

My birthday is in two days. This bicycle is my birthday present to myself.

Tuesday July 10

I go out to the garage and measure the gap between the saddle's two halves. It's 4 centimeters toward the front and back. In the middle, at its widest point, it's 4-1/2 centimeters.

I telephone Dr. Bruce. "The prostate is 3 to 4 centimeters in diameter," he says. "Your gap sounds wide enough to me."

"I'm still not going to ride it until after the PSA is drawn tomorrow. I rode a neighbor's bike without a split seat for an hour Sunday."

"By tomorrow any PSA elevation from that should be settled down. But this is uncharted territory. We don't know how much the PSA goes up and down in short periods of time, and we don't want to see any elevation of your PSA."

Wednesday July 11

I am 63 today. Eight months ago, on my brother's birthday, I found out that I had cancer. I'm worried about the PSA test today. But it has to be done.

The clinic coordinator is busy with an emergency when I arrive and can't get to me. I have a physical therapy appointment in half an hour, so I go there first, then come back to the hospital. I say a little prayer as the technician draws my blood.

It's been seven months since I began treatment and five months since I finished it. The radiation took exactly two months.

Thursday July 12

This morning I am apprehensive from the moment I wake up. I know Dr. Bruce will be gone today, and am damn nervous picking up the phone to call for the result.

"We don't want to see any elevation," he told me the other day.

All kinds of things are going through my head as I dial and wait. What if there is an elevation? Will I have to go through another battery of tests and treatments? I've chosen radiation, so surgery is no longer an option. On the other hand, even if there is a recurrence, prostate cancer usually grows very slowly. I think again of the roller coaster ride families of testicular cancer patients go through. I know what it's like. I'm on it.

I am cut off, nervously dial again, and speak with one of the nurses. "I'm calling for my PSA result. It was drawn yesterday."

Looking it up on the computer, she pauses. "Yours was down last time, wasn't it?"

"Yes," I say, but her question makes me apprehensive. Is it up now?

"It's 0.85," she says to my relief. "Down from 1.18."

I hang up and shout to Ilka. "I can ride my bike. The PSA's down."

"Thanks to me," she says. "If I hadn't bugged you, you wouldn't have gotten a PSA."

She may be right.

I phone our sons, David and Eric, and my brothers, Bob and Jack, but can't reach any of them. I call Todd and give him the good news.

Dr. Bruce said it would take a year and a half for the PSA to bottom out. It's definitely going in the right direction—down.

I go into the bathroom to comb my hair. "The last time you were here," I smirk to my image in the mirror, "you didn't know your PSA result. You do now."

Walking the dogs, I see our neighbor Jen across the street. "How're you?" she calls.

"Good," I say, "and all the better because my PSA is down."

"Wonderful," she says.

When I am back in the house, the phone rings. It is Mary, Don's wife.

"Yesterday, on my 63rd birthday, I had a PSA and it's down," I say.

"Congratulations and happy birthday," she says, "in that order."

"I should call it my PSA-day," I say.

She chuckles. "Thanks again for talking with Don and me before he made his decision. It sure helped."

Friday July 13

Larry phones. "After three months," he says, "I've finally decided on hormones and radiation. I start the hormones soon and will be on them three to five months, continuing them during radiation."

He chuckles. "My cholesterol hovers around 250 no matter what I do. I've tried dietary means to lower it, including soy bean products; cooked tomatoes; fatty omega-3 fish—salmon, mackerel, sardines, black cod; red wine; and selenium supplements. None of it lowered my cholesterol, but my PSA went from 5.5 to 5.0."

Wednesday July 19

I have an appointment with Dr. Bruce, who was gone last week. "Any sexual dysfunction?" he asks.

"I've never had that," I say, "during or after radiation."

"How are the bowels and urination?"

"No blood in stools for months. I go all night without getting up, and hold my urine better now than in several years."

He smiles. "You know, there really were beams coming out of that machine."

No rectal exam today. He wants me to return in three months for another examination and PSA.

Tuesday July 24

I receive an e-mail today from Larry:

Jim,

After numerous consultations/discussions and extensive literature research, I've finally decided on a treatment plan with my doctors, which starts today.

Here are the gory details. I'll be receiving hormone treatment under the care of a medical oncologist who refers to the treatment as androgen suppression. I'll get a Lupron shot in the butt monthly and take a pill (Casodex) a day for a period to be determined, prior to starting radiation treatment (Intensity Modulated Radiation Therapy, or IMRT).

Recent medical literature reports that for my condition (Gleason 7 was the key factor), receiving hormones prior to radiation decreases the probability of relapse by 50 percent,

> Intensity Modulated Radiation Therapy, or IMRT, is the latest form of external beam radiation therapy and has become the standard.

thereby increasing my probability of success to over 90 percent—which compares favorably to a predicted success rate for me of over 80 percent for surgery.

My PSA level should drop to near zero, and how fast it does determines when I'll start the radiation. If it's a rapid response I'll start radiation in a couple months, and if it's slow it could be five or six months, sometimes even longer. The faster the drop in PSA, the better the prognosis.

Other than the side effects (hot flashes, etc.), I should be pretty much normal during the hormone treatment. Once I start radiation I should continue to be pretty much normal, except for the added possibility of radiation fatigue. But I won't be able to travel as I will be getting zapped up in Santa

Monica/UCLA Med Center, Mondays through Fridays, for six to nine weeks. The schedule will be determined by my radiation oncologist who will take into consideration my response to the hormone treatment, among many other factors.

The hormones continue during radiation and conclude when the radiation ends. If all goes well I could be finished with the treatments by the end of November. After that, as you know, it will be a continual monitoring of my PSA level for evidence of recurrence. If I can make it for five years without relapse, then chances are good I've been cured—which is what I hope for both of us.

My thanks for your experience-based counsel.

Larry

Sunday August 12

Janice, an old friend, calls from San Francisco. I tell her about my prostate cancer.

"I didn't know you had that," she says. "But I'm very glad you chose radiation. If Bill and I had to deal with it, that's probably the way we'd go. Prostate cancer for men is what breast cancer is for women. So many options are available."

Wednesday August 22

Ilka tells me that two months after Don finished his radiation therapy his PSA was measured at 3.0.

"3.0?" I say. Then I remember him telling me this a couple of months ago. "Mine was lower than that about two months after radiation. It was 1.18."

"I didn't mention that to him," she says, "because I didn't want to worry him. I said yours was similar to his, and he said, 'Jim and I are just about the same with this disease.'"

At five months my PSA is 0.85, a number I'm so far very pleased about.

Thursday August 23

When I awake this morning I begin worrying I have steered Don to a treatment that might not be good for him. Perhaps surgery would have been better.

Wednesday August 29

Another e-mail from Larry:

> Hi Jim,
>
> How ya doing? I'm just into my second month of hormone therapy, and I think I'm doing OK. Prior to starting the hormones, my PSA had dropped from 5.8 to 4.9. My doctor wanted to know if I was taking saw palmetto or something like that, but I wasn't. I had started drinking green tea instead of coffee, taking a selenium supplement and eating more tomatoes and a lot more soy products : tofu, edamame and soy milk. He thinks maybe the soy products had a positive effect.
>
> I haven't gotten the results of last week's blood work, but if my PSA has dropped a lot then I'll probably start IMRT around late September—otherwise they'll wait another month or two. I go in after Labor Day to get the IMRT prep work done. I guess they have to do some measurements on me and calibrate their machines somehow.
>
> Larry

I think back on my planning session, now many months ago.

Friday August 31

Every time I ride my bike I think about the pressure that the seat, even though it's split, might be delivering to my prostate. Since I'm not over the hamstring injury, I need to bike. I can only hope I'm not in for an unpleasant surprise. If that should occur, Dr. Bruce said I would have to stop biking for a couple of weeks and get another PSA.

Friday September 7

Another e-mail from Larry:

> Jim,
>
> Eat more ketchup. Here's evidence that ketchup consumption does you good (I guess I should have eaten a lot more of it)— and ketchup on salmon may make you live forever!
>
> Larry

The e-mail contains two articles, the first extolling the virtues of lycopene, a chemical existing in copious amounts in tomato sauce. Lycopene appears not only to prevent prostate cancer, but to retard its progression if it's already present.

In a study done at the University of Illinois at Chicago, prostate cancer patients ate one tomato-based pasta dish per day for three weeks, each entrée containing 3/4 of a cup of tomato sauce. Over the three weeks, lycopene increased in the participants' blood and prostate tissue. Oxidation damage, which has been linked to cancer, decreased. The patients' PSA levels also dropped, suggesting that the number of cancer cells might have diminished.

The second article points out the virtues of consuming oily fish and the omega-3 fatty acids in them. It says omega-3 fatty acids might reduce the risk of colon and breast cancer, and that a recent Swedish study concludes that consuming oily fish might cut the risk of prostate cancer in half.

Monday October 8

I call Dr. Bruce's office and schedule an appointment for a PSA test on Thursday the 17th. He's in Australia until later this month. I'm somewhat nervous about the PSA, partly because I've been riding the bike almost every day for three months.

Monday October 15

I change my appointment from Thursday the 17th to Wednesday the 16th because we close on a new home mortgage on Friday and I don't want to risk getting bad news and not having time to discuss it with an oncologist.

Wednesday October 17

I go to the hospital for my PSA blood test. It's so crowded when I get there I have to wait until another patient pulls out to get a parking space. This has never happened before. The waiting room is crowded, too. Glancing about at the patients and their families, I am relieved to be a graduate of cancer treatment (hopefully a graduate, if all keeps going well) rather than an active participant. You can tell who the patients are. Many look sick, depleted, and rundown.

Before going to the lab I speak to the clinic coordinator. "In Dr. Bruce's absence, can I call the department tomorrow for the test result?"

"Yes," she says, "but it might not be available before noon."

I go to the lab, which is also busy. As I wait, a man comes in and sits down beside me. I've seen him earlier in the oncology waiting room. He looks the right age to be a prostate patient, and I think he's probably sitting there with a full bladder. I am glad I'm not in his shoes anymore. A radiation therapist arrives to take him back for treatment, telling him that he will return here afterwards.

A man and a woman are here with a tiny baby, the man feeding the baby with an eye dropper. The baby is taken in to have some blood drawn, and a few minutes later the technician comes out with a small tube of blood. I wonder what disease that tiny patient has.

Later, as a technician is drawing my blood, I ask whether he is taking the blood for a PSA test (I'm just checking), and he says yes.

Thursday October 18

Awaiting my PSA result, I am less nervous than I was back in July. I guess I'm more confident about the results now.

I take the dogs out for a walk. When I come back to my computer, a note from Ilka is sitting on it. The note reads:

> PSA Results
> 1.18 April
> 0.85 July
> 0.55 Oct

Still going down despite my biking. That question is answered. And the radiation therapy seems to have succeeded.
"Hey, great!" I call to Ilka. "The hospital phoned?"
"Yes," she says. "I thought you'd like that result."

I call my brother Jack, my cousin Ellen, our sons Eric and David, and our friends Don, Todd, and Mark. All are pleased. As am I.

I call Larry in Los Angeles. "In an hour," he says, "I'm going in to be measured and prepped for radiation, which will start in a week."
"It's your planning session," I say.
"They're gonna tattoo me where the sun don't shine."
"Your crosshatches."
"I'm on hormones and my sex life has gone away, but I haven't had hot flashes or other side effects. A month ago my PSA was down to 0.27 from the hormones, maybe dietary changes, too."

Later David phones back. "Those prostate cells must be all shriveled up down there."

I ride my bike around the lake, and for the first time I don't worry about my PSA.

Tuesday October 23

The first anniversary of my learning that I have prostate cancer.

Wednesday October 24

I see Dr. Bruce for a check-up. I'm not nervous because I already know the PSA result.

"Your score of 0.55 is very good," he says. "But I can't tell you you're out of the woods yet."

"I've heard about IMRT," I say. "A friend in Los Angeles is having it."

"Intensity Modulated Radiation Therapy, the most advanced form of conformal radiation treatment. We started using it here when you were halfway through your treatments. I considered switching you to it, but there's a learning curve. Your brother's a friend and you're a doctor. I think problems can arise when a physician treats another physician, because you try to do something extra, do too much. So I didn't change anything."

"And my PSA is coming down."

"Yes, but there's a chance it could go back up. We used to think that if it rose on three consecutive occasions, it meant a recurrence of tumor. But that perception's changing because we've learned in seed patients it can rise and go back down again."

"Has anything changed between urologists and oncologists regarding prostate cancer treatment?"

"No, it will take a long time."

Friday October 26

During breakfast our handyman mentions that his father died of prostate cancer at age 77. "He was a high school teacher in a small town, and was close friends with the local doctor. Because of their friendship, I suspect the doctor never gave my dad a thorough exam. By the time the cancer was found it was too late. He lived four more years. I moved in and took care of him toward the end."

"The disease had probably been there for some years," I say, "perhaps as many as 20. Prostate cancer is usually slow-growing."

Thursday November 1

Got this e-mail from Larry:

> Jim,
>
> My PSA is down to 0.18 (4.8 prior at start of hormone treatment, 0.27 after first month). After a second month of hormones I've started radiation treatment. 8:00 a.m. every day except weekends and holidays. I experienced minor nausea after yesterday's zapping—also had minor "hot flashes," which I never had while only getting hormone therapy. The hormone and radiation treatments should be completed just before Christmas. What's your latest PSA?
>
> Larry

I send the result, and say:

> It feels good being at the other end of those radiation treatments, and you soon will be.

Thursday November 8

Don calls. "I finished radiation seven months ago, and my PSA has dropped to 0.96. I'm pretty happy about that. Dr. Bruce felt my prostate and said it was better, softer, smaller, more normal."

"Any residuals from the radiation?" I ask.

"My stools are softer than before treatment, and I have more urgency to empty the bowel. I think it's from lingering rectal irritation. I had no decrease in potency during or after treatment, but have had some blood in the semen, which is lessening. Dr. Bruce said this wasn't common but does happen and should go away. Overall I'm very happy with the treatment."

Now I'm glad I steered him toward radiation after all.

Saturday November 10

Now I'm going to climb up onto my soap box. (Can you see me gesturing, a finger jutting skyward?) Ilka and I socialize with lots of people, but over the last year how many have called to see how I'm doing?

Damn few. I recently phoned one friend to congratulate his wife on an honor she'd received. "I've thought about calling you," he said, "but just didn't get around to it."

People aren't intentionally inconsiderate. We all live busy lives and—out of sight, out of mind. Who wants to call someone who will make us feel depressed because they're not doing well? I don't.

But shame on us, all of us. Know what? We don't think it's going to happen to us. I didn't think it would happen to me. But it did, and I've learned a few things. I'll pay more attention to people not doing well, who are out of circulation, out of the loop. That's when they need friends most.

Saturday November 17

I remember discussing prostate surgery with the urologist last year and thinking, mistakes are made in medicine. A physician acquaintance of mine once operated on the wrong hip.

Well, in the mail today I get my latest copy of *Orthopedics Today*. Here's the headline: "Wrong-site hand surgery rate: higher than previous estimates." In a survey of 1,050 hand surgeons, almost 20 percent reported performing surgery on the wrong site at least once. Seven percent of these unnecessary surgeries resulted in permanent disability.

Mistakes happen. A patient must stay as alert and aware as possible, and communicate assertively with health care providers.

Sunday November 18

Brunch with Carol and Phil. I speak privately with Phil, who's 76 years old.

"Your PSA is high, isn't it?" I ask.

"It's 27," he says. "I've had three biopsies, and they were all negative. I'm not having any more." He grins. "My prostate must look like Swiss cheese. I asked a friend, a urologist, how it could be so high. 'You probably have cancer they didn't find,' he told me."

At Phil's age the treatment would doubtless be watchful waiting anyway.

Driving home in the car I switch on the radio. The music is very familiar—the composition I listened to over and over while being radiated.

"Help me hear what the title of this is," I tell Ilka. "I know it's a Brandenburg Concerto, I just can't remember which one."

When the music ends, the announcer gives the title: Bach's Brandenburg Concerto No. 3.

My brother Jack had suggested I listen to music during radiation. "Make it something you don't like, because in the future you'll probably associate that music with bad memories."

That didn't happen. The music sounds wonderful to me.

Wednesday December 12

At 8:45 a.m. I phone Radiation Oncology, and the clinic coordinator answers.

"My PSA was drawn yesterday," I say. "I'm calling for the result."

"I'm not actually sure it's ready," she says, and puts me on hold. "Here it is, 0.37, down from 0.55 last time."

I hang up and tell Ilka.

"It keeps going down," she says.

It does, and lets keep it that way.

I see Dr. Bruce in his office. "That's a very good, low number," he says.

"Last time you told me I wasn't out of the woods yet," I say. "When will I be?"

He looks at me. "In 15 years. We can't call it a cure from cancer until you've lived 15 years after treatment. But with a PSA below 1.0, your chances are very good."

"Is that 15 years for all cancers or just prostate cancer?"

"Prostate, because it's usually a slow-growing tumor. For most cancers, including breast cancer, we call it a cure after five years. But even that's changing, since some breast cancers can recur after five years. The 15-year figure for prostate cancer is my standard."

"Assuming all goes well, how long will I be followed with examinations and PSA tests?"

"The rest of your life."

"Let's hope that's a long time."

AFTERWORD

In preparation for publishing this book, I contacted several of the men with prostate cancer whom I mention in my journal. I wanted to find out how their cases had progressed over time and, if they had it to do all over again, what treatment or treatments they would choose.

•   •   •

One friend, whose major problem after prostate cancer surgery was impotence, is now 75 years old. "Nine years ago," he says, "I had a transperineal prostatectomy, an operation done through the space between the scrotum and anus, which resulted in complete erectile dysfunction. I've had mild results with a vacuum pump, but not a satisfactory erection. I've tried Viagra, but it didn't work, and the last time I had intercourse was the night before surgery."

Prior to surgery his PSA went from 18 to 38, and he had prostate biopsies every six months until the cancer was finally discovered. "In those days," he says, "the PSA test wasn't covered by insurance, but surgery was, and the insurance company couldn't start paying fast enough when my cancer was discovered. I think many men died of prostate cancer because insurance didn't pay for the PSA and they didn't get the test. In my work as a minister I saw many people die, and dying of prostate cancer is one of the worst ways to go."

He works out without a urinary pad, but if he bends at the waist a lot, he leaks urine. If he is going to have a few drinks or play a long round of golf, he will also wear a pad.

He's had a PSA every year since surgery, and it's remained stable all this time, a recent reading being less than 0.1.

"What would you do if you had it to do over again?" I ask.

"Surgery!" he replies emphatically. "I think the surgeon saved my life. He followed my disease all along and thought it was a risk to leave anything inside. I'm fine now, cancer-free as far as I know. By the way, I realize you've changed peoples' names in this book, but if you want to use mine, go ahead. I'm not ashamed of anything. I'm a champion of this cause, of surgery. The impotence used to bother me, but one accommodates to getting older."

• • •

Larry in Los Angeles is now 65 years old. He finished his hormones and external beam radiation therapy almost three years ago. His Gleason score before he began treatment was 7 and his PSA was 5.8. Three months before radiation he started taking Lupron and Casodex, anti-testosterone hormones. Then he underwent Intensity Modulated Radiation Therapy (IMRT) five days a week for nine weeks, continuing the hormones a month after the radiation stopped.

"During treatment," he says, "I sometimes had pain with a bowel movement, a few times bad, and blood, sometimes quite a bit, on the toilet paper but never in the toilet bowl. I occasionally still have blood on the tissue."

"Did you have radiation fatigue?" I ask.

"Halfway through treatment it came on, but I'd take a 30-minute nap and be fine again. About the same time I stopped playing tennis because of fatigue. In fact the last time I played during treatment I had to quit halfway through the match, but I started playing again six weeks after therapy."

"How about erectile dysfunction?"

"I had no erections during treatment, presumably because of the hormones. My erections returned three months after the hormones ended and are adequate but not what they used to be. I've got Viagra but haven't needed to use it."

"What's your most recent PSA?"

"That's fluctuated. A year ago it shot up from 0.4 to 1.4, and my oncologist said that's not good and suggested another biopsy, but we decided to wait. A month later it was 0.8, after another month 0.6, and three months later it was back down to 0.4. The latest one was 0.48."

"Incontinence?"

He responds in his usual blunt fashion. "I've never had that or urinary problems, but for several months in the past year I've had rectal urgency. I didn't dare fart because I thought I'd crap in my pants. That's not still happening, but my bowel habits have changed from every morning like a clock to almost a random thing, and not even every day, and usually not with urgency."

"If you had to do it all over again, what would you do?"

"My choice came down to surgery versus hormones and radiation. I'd probably do what I did, but I have friends who had surgery and seem to be doing okay."

• • •

The man who was taking Lupron to shut down his testosterone is now 84 years old.

"The first surgeon I saw was related to Dracula," he says. "Wanted me to give two or three pints of blood before surgery because they lose a lot during the operation. I wasn't ready to go under the knife and dodged the issue for a while. It's a male disease, and my doctors were all male, but they treated it like a tennis match. I saw a doctor in Florida who put me on Lupron, and my PSA went to zero. Then he put the seeds in, but they didn't get the job done. After a couple of years my PSA shot up to 7 or 8. I've been on the hormone

Casodex for the last two or three years, and I still have prostate cancer, but I'm 84 and I don't want anything else done.

"If I had it to do over again," he says, "I'd probably do the same thing. No surgery. I've had too many friends go under the knife without successful conclusions."

His PSA now is 7.5. He's had no incontinence, but also no erections for a long time. "You could put me in a room full of naked women," he says, "and I'd probably just walk out the door."

• • •

Fred, the financial analyst, works in a large eastern city. "Six years ago my PSA went from 4 to 8 or 9," he says. "I had a biopsy and scan, and my local urologist recommended surgery."

Seeking the best treatment, he went to one of the country's urologic centers of excellence, where he had a nerve-sparing radical prostatectomy. As far as the cancer goes, his results were good: his PSA is now practically zero, and he considers himself disease-free.

"The nursing care there was great," he says, "but the a urologist was a cold fish. Wearing the catheter was awful, and I got a minor infection from it. I was assured that after surgery I wouldn't have trouble with sexual function, yet the surgery ruined my sex life. I haven't had an erection since and never will. Over the years my wife and I had been having fewer sexual encounters, and this did nothing to help that situation. And it's played havoc with my head, because I'm still interested in sex, yet unable to perform."

"Any incontinence?" I ask.

"I guess you'd call it stress incontinence. Playing tennis I get a little wet, but I also sweat a lot, and I don't wear a pad."

"If you had it to do over again, what would you do?"

"Over the past six years three or four men with prostate cancer have called me asking what to do. I've said consider the seeds, because there's a better chance of retaining potency than with prostatectomy. Surgery's certainly not my first choice."

• • •

The next man, who is 66 years old, isn't mentioned in my journal because I didn't meet him until after it was written. Having already chosen to be treated by external beam radiation, he said that reading my journal in manuscript form was of immeasurable help to him. "It took me through every step of the process, and I knew exactly what would happen beforehand."

This man's PSA before he began treatment was in the mid-20s and his Gleason score was 7. Because of these relatively high numbers, he first underwent laparoscopic exploration and biopsy of the seminal vesicles, prostate, and lymph nodes to determine whether the cancer had spread outside the prostate gland.

"Cancer was found in the seminal vesicles and prostate," he says, "but not in the lymph nodes. I was given the hormone Lupron for three months before treatment, had external beam radiation, and continued Lupron for two years afterwards.

"During radiation I had marked urgency of bowel and diarrhea, which continues intermittently. I take an anti-diarrheal as needed, and the symptoms are controlled. I had no urinary incontinence during or after treatment, but I did experience fatigue during radiation. The fatigue could have been caused by the Lupron, however."

While taking Lupron he could not achieve an erection, and that's still more or less true today. "I was told," he says, "that it would take 6 to 12 months before the effects of the hormone were out of my system, and I've been off it for 8 months. On a scale of 1 to 10, my erections are a 2. I've tried Viagra and one other medication without great results, and haven't tried the third. My testosterone level had been in the 20s and was recently up to 125, which is still below normal."

His PSA has been less than 0.05 for two years. When I ask what he would do if he could start all over again, he says, "I wouldn't change a thing."

• • •

The old family friend who experienced prominent fatigue during external beam radiation and couldn't do more than go to therapy and come home and lie on the couch finished treatment five years ago. His most recent PSA was 0.06. He was 80 years old when diagnosed with prostate cancer. "I saw my urologist," he says, "and he laid out all the choices of treatment. He did *not* encourage me to have surgery. I chose external beam radiation."

The doctor warned him that he would have rectal tenderness, diarrhea, and fatigue. "I decided to pamper myself and stayed in bed, sleeping a great deal and leading a very quiet life. I did have some rectal tenderness but no diarrhea. I drove myself to treatment five days a week for eight weeks. I found myself intrigued by the massive machines and appreciating the technicians handling me."

I ask him about incontinence. "When I'm out and about, I occasionally wear a Kleenex in my shorts, and sometimes there's a drip, but I don't use a diaper."

When asked what treatment he would choose if he had it to do over again, he says, "Exactly what I did."

"How bad was the radiation fatigue?" I ask.

"It was bad to me," he says, "but then I was a premature baby, and I've been tired since I was born."

• • •

Don, together with his wife, Mary, decided on external beam radiation after consulting with me and my wife. His pre-treatment PSA was 8. He's now 69 years old, and three years after therapy his PSA is 1.13.

"Throughout radiation, the fiber in my diet caused loose stools, and this was treated with an over-the-counter anti-diarrheal," he says. "For almost a year following radiation, the problem continued, but now I'm almost back to normal. During treatment I had mild pain on urination and decreased flow, both of which have improved with medication. I had no radiation fatigue. After treatment I had slight incontinence, but currently my urination is fine. For six months after treatment I had a small amount of blood in my sperm, but that's back to normal, too."

Asked about erectile function, he says things are "working fine," and when asked what treatment he would choose if he had it to do over again, he says "the same thing I did."

• • •

Called one of his "successes" by the urologist who did his radical prostatectomy seven years ago, Steve had a pre-operative PSA between 4 and 5 and a Gleason score of 5.

Now, at age 71, he's an active person, sometimes playing tennis twice a day. "I did that today," he said when we talked. "In singles tennis I still wear a small pad because of minor urine leakage. If I have a big dinner and take a walk in the evening, or have a full stomach and haven't had a bowel movement, or lean forward and there's pressure against the bladder, I can have seepage.

"If I had it to do over again, I'd ask more questions about postoperative erectile function. The surgery affected mine. It's not as good as it once was, and I'm disappointed about that, but I understand that this is part of the procedure. No promises were made. I knew I might be in this position. I don't think about it that much anymore. I just live with it. I have a PSA twice a year, and it's hardly measurable. My mind's at ease as long as the PSA stays down, and I recommend my urologist highly."

• • •

And what about me? Now, over four years after radiation therapy, my PSA is 0.14.

I haven't had the dreaded complications of prostate cancer treatment: impotence and incontinence. In recent months I've occasionally had small amounts of blood in my urine and semen, which have been interpreted as rare late side effects of radiation. My radiation was 3D-CRT. With the newest form of external beam radiation—IMRT—there may be less chance of such side effects.

If I had it to do over again? I'd do just what I did.

GLOSSARY

3-D radiation therapy (3D-CRT): Radiation therapy designed to avoid radiation injury to normal tissues surrounding a tumor, while concentrating energy as accurately as possible on the tumor itself.

BAT (B-mode Acquisition and Targeting): ultrasound localizer, used to locate the exact region to be radiated.

benign: Tissue not having the elements of cancer, having cells which divide in an orderly fashion.

biopsy: Surgical removal of tissue for examination under a microscope. A needle biopsy is performed with a needle; an open biopsy is done through an incision.

bladder: Reservoir for urine, which it receives from the kidneys and releases into the urethra.

brachytherapy: Placing radioactivity in or near a targeted area, frequently a tumor. With prostate cancer, tiny radioactive seeds are implanted in the gland to impart concentrated, localized radiation.

The seeds are metal-encapsulated pellets containing the radioisotope Iodine-125 or Palladium-103. A seed is about 1/8th of an inch long and has the thickness of a paper clip. The number implanted varies from approximately 50 to 100.

cancer: Malignant abnormality of cells causing them to multiply and grow uncontrollably.

capsule: Membranous layer surrounding an organ or part.

cells: Minute, independently operating units composing the structure of all organisms.

colonoscopy: Colon examination with a colonoscope to search for cancer and biopsy suspicious tissue.

conformal radiation therapy (3D-CRT): Radiation therapy designed to avoid radiation injury to tissue surrounding a tumor, while concentrating energy as accurately as possible on the tumor itself.

cryotherapy (cryosurgery, cryoablation): Use of subfreezing temperatures to affect a tissue structure or cell. For example, freezing prostatic tissue to kill cells.

digital rectal exam (DRE): Examination in which the examiner's lubricated, gloved finger is inserted into the rectum to examine the rectum and prostate gland.

Gleason score: Score given by a pathologist after examining specimens of a prostate gland, or the entire gland, under a microscope. The score rates the aggressiveness of the prostate cancer cells.

impotence: Also known as erectile dysfunction, inability to maintain an erection of sufficient firmness to engage in penetrative sex.

incontinence, urinary: Inability to hold urine in the bladder.

malignant: Tissue having the elements of cancer with cells dividing in an uncontrolled fashion.

metastasis: 1. Spread of cancer from its original site to another part of the body; 2. A portion of a cancerous tumor that has spread from its original site to another part of the body.

metastasize: To spread from an original site to another part of the body (referring to cancer).

prostate: Small gland in males lying behind the pubic bone, above the base of the penis, below the bladder, and in front of the rectum. Its function is to produce a portion of the fluid of the ejaculate.

prostate cancer: Cancer of the prostate gland, almost always adenocarcinoma.

prostatectomy: Surgical removal of the prostate gland.

prostatitis: Inflammation or infection of the prostate gland.

prostate-specific antigen (PSA): Enzyme secreted by prostate cells. The PSA blood test is widely used to screen for prostate cancer.

semen: Liquid ejaculate made up of sperm and fluid (from accessory glands) which nourishes and propels the sperm.

seminal vesicles: Pair of small organs lying adjacent to the prostate and contributing to fluid production for semen.

stricture: Narrowing of a body passage, especially a tube or canal, restricting flow through the tube.

tumor: Abnormal mass or growth, either non-cancerous or cancerous.

urethra: Tube carrying urine from the bladder to the outside. In the male it also carries semen.

Websites

The websites listed below are respected, dependable resources for information on prostate cancer. Be aware, however, that some information posted on the Internet is inaccurate, biased, or deliberately misleading. Even when factual, the information may not be appropriate for your particular case. Consult with your physician before acting on any medical advice you find on the Internet.

For further information on prostate cancer, visit Dr. James Priest's website at www.jamespriest.com.

American Cancer Society: www.cancer.org

American Foundation for Urologic Disease: www.afud.org

CancerSource.com: www.cancersource.com

Hisandherhealth.com: www.hisandherhealth.com

James Buchanan Brady Urological Institute, Johns Hopkins
Medicine: www.urology.jhu.edu

Mayo Clinic: www.mayoclinic.com

National Cancer Institute, U.S. National Institutes of Health: www.cancer.gov

National Prostate Cancer Coalition: www.pcacoalition.org

PSA Rising: www.psa-rising.com

Us TOO International: www.ustoo.com

WebMD Health: my.webmd.com

Books

Bostwick, David G., M.D., MBA, E. David Crawford, M.D., Celestia S. Higano, M.D., and Mack Roach III, M.D., eds. *American Cancer Society's Complete Guide to Prostate Cancer*. Atlanta: American Cancer Society, 2005.

Scardino, Peter T., M.D., and Judith Kelman. *Dr. Peter Scardino's Prostate Book*. New York: Avery, 2005.

Walsh, Patrick C., M.D., and Janet Farrar Worthington. *Dr. Patrick Walsh's Guide to Surviving Prostate Cancer*. New York: Warner Books, 2001.

3D simulation, 51
3D conformal external beam
    radiation (3D-CRT), 22, 23,
    34, 38–40, 52, 53, 70, 85,
    125, 126, 130, 132, 134, 157,
    159. *See also* external beam
    radiation.

adrenal gland, 73
alternative medicine, 16, 134, 135
analgesic, 84
androgen suppression, 73, 139
anesthesia/anesthetic, 18, 60, 111
antibiotic, 1, 2, 19, 104
antibody, 121
antigen. *See* prostate-specific
    antigen.
antioxidant, 108
anus, 151
avascular necrosis, 131

BAT ultrasound machine, 22, 23,
    53, 56, 58, 64, 70, 77, 85, 125,
    159
benign, 25, 31, 50, 109, 159
benign prostatic hyperplasia
    (BPH), 12, 83, 110, 115
biological therapy, 42
biopsy, 2, 12, 16, 17, 18–19,
    24–25, 36, 42, 52, 71, 79, 84,
    90, 112, 113, 118, 125, 129,
    148, 151, 153, 154, 155, 159,
    160
bladder, 2, 7, 10, 23, 36, 38, 39,
    51, 55, 56, 57, 58, 59, 62, 63,
    66, 68, 70, 71, 74, 75, 76, 82,
    83, 86, 87, 88, 89, 91, 92, 93,
    95, 96–97, 100, 101, 123,
    126, 143, 157, 159, 161, 162;
    infection of, 116; inflamma-
    tion of, 130; irritation of, 33,
    51, 68, 69. 81, 86, 98

bladder urgency. *See* urgency.
bladder frequency. *See* frequency.
blood-thinning medication, 18
bone scan, 4, 8, 10, 15, 59, 95
bowel frequency. *See* frequency.
bowel movement, pain or difficulty with. *See* rectal pain.
bowel urgency. *See* urgency.
brachytherapy, 48, 60–61,
90–91, 102, 132, 159. *See also*
radioactive seeds.

cancer cell, 2, 5, 16, 24–25,
30–31, 36, 45, 53, 54, 59, 67,
71, 72–73, 79, 90, 109, 113,
120, 121, 142, 160, 161
capsule (lining of the prostate),
34, 160
Casodex, 139, 152, 154
catheter, 2, 4, 16, 17, 36, 60, 79,
110, 120, 154
chemotherapy, 42, 75, 91, 95
Cialis, 103
colonoscopy, 1, 28, 29, 52, 112,
160
complementary medicine,
114–115
complication, 16, 34, 35, 36, 43,
49, 102, 122; bladder/uri-
nary, 23, 34, 35, 38, 61;
bowel/rectal, 23, 34, 38, 61;
of brachytherapy (radioactive seeds), 34, 40, 60–61,
96; of cryotherapy, 78, 80,
91; of external beam

radiation, 23, 34, 38, 40, 41,
49, 52, 64, 107, 110, 122, 157;
of hormonal therapy, 73; of
needle biopsy, 18; of prostate
surgery, 2, 4, 5, 16, 34, 37, 40,
67, 76, 96, 107, 110, 111, 112,
113, 116, 120, 125. *See also* side
effect.
contraction (of urethral sphincter), 63, 64, 69, 86, 94
crosshatch, 50, 58, 65, 68, 99,
144
cryoablation. See cryotherapy.
cryoprobe, 79
cryosurgery. See cryotherapy.
cryotherapy, 14, 72, 78–80, 91,
102, 114, 129, 132, 160
cure rate, 4, 16, 136, 140
cystitis, 130

digital rectal exam (DRE), 12–13,
18, 24, 38, 84, 138, 160
DNA, 30–31, 54
dosimetrist, 51, 55

ejaculation, 7, 12, 127
enlargement of the prostate. *See*
benign prostatic hyperplasia.
enzyme, 12, 161
erectile dysfunction. *See* impotence.
estrogen, 73
external beam radiation, 14, 21,
22, 23, 26, 27, 29, 32, 33,

34–35, 38, 40, 41, 47, 49, 53, 54, 60, 70, 72, 78, 79, 81, 88, 90, 91, 102, 113, 118, 120, 125, 129–130, 132, 134–135, 139, 152, 155, 156, 157. *See also* 3D conformal external beam radiation; complication; radiation therapy.

false negative, 14
false positive, 14
FDA, 114
fiber, 88, 92, 104, 106, 112, 117, 156
field (of radiation), 75, 83, 86
fish oil, 108–109, 138, 142
fistula, 80, 91
Flomax, 87
free radical, 54
frequency, bladder/urinary, 34, 61, 87, 89, 100, 101, 122; bowel/rectal, 87, 89

gene therapy, 29, 46, 121
general anesthesia, 60
genes/genetics, 29, 31, 46, 54, 121
gland. *See* adrenal gland; lymph node; prostate gland.
Gleason score, 2, 16, 24–25, 27, 60, 84, 113, 115, 125, 128, 129, 134, 135, 139, 152, 155, 157, 160

half-life (of radioactive isotopes), 8, 60
herbal medicine, 114–115
hesitancy (on starting urination), 112
hormonal treatment (for prostate cancer), 17, 42, 72–73, 78, 84, 90–91
hormone, 7
hot flash, 27, 72, 139, 144, 146

immune system, 30, 106
immunotherapy, 42, 114, 121
implant for treating impotence, 16, 103; for treating incontinence, 26, 48
implantation of radiative seeds (brachytherapy), 14, 20, 28, 34, 60–61, 78, 159–160
impotence, as a complication of treatment for prostate cancer, 2, 4, 16, 34, 37, 40, 49, 57, 61, 67, 72, 76, 80, 82, 84, 102–103, 107, 116, 120, 121, 125, 130, 132, 151, 152, 153, 157, 160; treatments for, 16, 57, 76, 103, 116
incontinence (urinary), as a complication of treatment for prostate cancer, 2, 4, 5, 16, 23, 26–27, 34, 36–37, 38, 40, 48–49, 57, 61, 67, 71, 76, 79–80, 82, 84, 91, 107, 110, 120, 121, 125, 127, 153, 154, 155, 156, 157, 161; stress, 38, 154

infection, 32, 35, 36–37, 67; from
    needle biopsy of prostate,
    18–19; of bladder, 4, 12, 16,
    116, 154; of prostate gland, 1,
    12, 161
inflammation of bladder (cysti-
    tis), 130; of prostate gland
    (prostatitis), 1, 161; of rec-
    tum (proctitis), 130
Intensity Modulated Radiation
    Therapy (IMRT), 40, 120,
    139, 141, 145, 152, 157
Iodine-125, 60, 160. *See also*
    radioactive isotope.
isotope. *See* radioactive isotope.

laparoscopic prostatectomy, 16,
    120–121
Levitra, 103
luteinizing hormone-releasing
    hormone analog (LHRH), 73.
    See also Lupron; Zoladex.
local anesthetic, 18
localized cancer, 22, 60, 78, 91,
    121
lumbar spine, 15
Lupron, 22, 27, 73, 128, 139, 152,
    153, 155. *See also* hormonal
    treatment.
lycopene, 108–109, 142
lymph node, 30, 46, 90, 155
lymphatics, 30
lymphoid tissue, 106

malignant (cancerous) cell, 24,
    25, 30–31, 53, 109, 160, 161
margin (around prostate gland),
    23, 79
metastasis, 30, 60, 108, 161
microscope, examination of cells
    under, 2, 7, 16, 18, 24–25, 31,
    71, 159, 160
minimally invasive surgery. *See*
    laparoscopic prostatectomy.

needle biopsy (of prostate
    gland), 12, 18–19, 159. *See
    also* biopsy.
nerve-sparing surgery, 66, 110,
    154. *See also* radical prostatec-
    tomy; surgery.
nodule, 38, 122

oily fish. *See* fish oil.
omega-3 fatty acids. *See* fish oil.
oncologist, 3, 20, 21, 22, 23, 28,
    33, 38, 42–43, 47, 49, 55, 81,
    96, 97, 100, 125, 126, 127,
    129, 134, 139, 140, 143, 145,
    153
open biopsy (of prostate gland),
    159. *See also* biopsy.
open prostatectomy, 120. *See also*
    radical prostatectomy; sur-
    gery.
orchiectomy, 73
orthopedics, 8, 11
orthopedist, 5, 50, 112, 131

Palladium-103, 60, 160. *See also* radioactive isotope.

palliative care, 90–91

pathologist, 7, 18, 24, 31, 160

pathology, 24, 129

PC-SPES, 114

pelvis, 10, 15, 80, 91, 98, 131, 133, 134

penis, 7, 79, 103, 122, 161

polyp, 29, 52

proctitis, 130

prostate gland, 7, 12, 22, 38, 54, 71, 72, 102, 122, 147, 148, 160, 161; biopsy of, 2, 12, 16, 17, 18–19, 24–25, 36, 42, 71, 79, 84, 90, 112, 113, 118, 125, 129, 148, 151, 153, 154, 155, 159; effects of biking on, 135, 136, 142; enlargement of (benign prostatic hyperplasia), 12, 83, 110, 115; examining digitally (digital rectal exam), 12–13, 18, 24, 38, 84, 138, 160; freezing of (cryotherapy), 14, 72, 78–80, 91, 102, 114, 129, 132, 160; *illustration*, 6; implanting radioactive seeds in (brachytherapy), 20, 21, 48, 60–61, 90–91, 102, 132, 159; infection/inflammation of (prostatitis), 1, 12, 62, 104, 161; lining of (capsule), 34, 160; locating position of (for radiation), 22–23, 56, 57, 58, 63, 64, 69; radiation of (external beam radiation), 14, 21, 22, 23, 26, 27, 29, 32, 33, 34–35, 38, 40, 41, 47, 49, 53, 54, 60, 70, 72, 78, 79, 81, 88, 90, 91, 102, 113, 118, 120, 125, 129–130, 132, 134–135, 139, 152, 155, 156, 157; surgical removal of (prostatectomy), 2, 4, 5, 15, 16, 17, 23, 26, 27, 29, 32, 33, 34, 34, 36–37, 39, 40, 42, 43, 48, 49, 51, 52, 53, 57, 61, 62, 66–67, 71, 72, 74, 79, 81, 84, 90, 91, 96, 102, 103, 107, 110, 111, 112, 113, 116, 117, 118, 120, 122, 125, 126, 127, 129, 130, 132, 134, 135, 137, 139, 141, 148, 151, 152, 153, 154, 155, 156, 157, 161

prostate bed, 90

prostatectomy. *See* surgery.

prostate-specific antigen (PSA), 12–13, 161. *See also* PSA test.

prostatitis, 1, 12, 62, 104, 161

proton beam radiation, 120

PSA test, 1, 2, 4, 7, 12–14, 18, 19, 26, 27, 28, 32, 39, 42, 60, 61, 62, 84, 85, 90–91, 98, 109, 113, 115, 118, 119, 122, 123, 124, 126, 127, 129, 130, 131, 134, 135, 136, 137, 138, 139, 140, 141, 142, 143, 144, 145, 146, 147, 148, 149, 151, 152, 153, 154, 155, 156, 157, 161

pubic bone, 7, 50, 70, 161

pump, for treating erectile dysfunction, 37, 76, 103, 151; for treating urinary incontinence, 26–27, 48

rad, 85

radiation fatigue, 51, 59, 68, 69, 77, 83, 89, 94, 104, 139, 152, 156

radiation oncologist, 20, 21, 22, 23, 28, 42–43, 47, 49, 52, 55, 96, 97, 100, 125, 126, 129, 140. *See also* oncologist.

radiation therapist, 50, 56, 58, 143

radiation therapy, 2, 14, 16, 17, 21, 22, 23, 26, 27, 29, 32, 33, 34, 35, 38, 39, 40, 41, 42, 43, 44, 45, 47, 49, 50, 51, 52, 53, 54–55, 56, 57, 59, 60–61, 63, 64, 65, 68, 69, 70, 72, 74, 75, 76, 77, 78, 79, 80, 81, 82, 83, 84, 85, 86, 87, 88, 89, 90–91, 92, 93, 94, 96–97, 98, 99, 100, 102, 106, 107, 110, 112, 113, 114, 118–120, 122, 123, 125, 126, 127, 128, 129, 130, 131, 132, 134, 135, 138, 139, 140, 144, 146, 147, 148, 149, 145, 152, 153, 155, 156, 157, 159, 160. *See also* 3D conformal external beam radiation; brachytherapy; external beam radiation;

Intensity Modulated Radiation Therapy (IMRT); radioactive seeds.

radical prostatectomy, 2, 15, 21, 22, 34, 39, 40, 53, 66–67, 76, 80, 81, 96, 102, 103, 113, 120, 129, 154, 157. *See also* surgery.

radioactive dye, 8, 9, 10

radioactive isotope, 8, 9, 10, 60, 160

radioactive seeds, 14, 20, 21, 54, 60–61, 78, 90–91, 96, 159. *See also* brachytherapy.

radioactivity, 9, 60, 159

radioisotope. *See* radioactive isotope.

radiologist, 15

radiotherapy. *See* radiation therapy.

rectal frequency. *See* frequency.

rectal pain, 34, 61, 98, 152

rectal probe, 2, 18, 79

rectal urgency. *See* urgency.

rectum, 7, 18, 23, 24, 38, 51, 55, 68, 79, 80, 88, 91, 96–97, 98, 130, 160, 161

recurrence (of cancer), 33, 35, 39, 49, 78, 80, 91, 97, 132, 137, 140, 145, 149

regional (site of cancer), 22

removal of the prostate. *See* surgery.

robotic-laparoscopic prostatectomy, 120-121

salvage surgery, 16, 91

saw palmetto, 114–115, 141

screening (for cancer), 1, 13, 18, 84, 161

scrotum, 151

seeds. *See* radioactive seeds.

selenium, 5, 16, 32, 114, 138, 141

semen, 7, 12, 38, 147, 157, 161, 162

seminal vesicle, 83, 155, 161

serum marker, 123

sex, 1, 2, 16, 17, 40, 49, 57, 61, 70, 80, 82, 98, 103, 110, 111, 116, 122, 130, 138, 144, 154, 160

sexual dysfunction. *See* impotence.

side effect, 43, 49, 116, 122; of hormones, 139, 144; of laparoscopic prostatectomy, 121; of radiation therapy, 33, 51, 52, 68, 85, 96–97, 98, 104, 113, 127, 130, 157; of prostate surgery, 33; of selenium, 114; of vitamin E, 109. *See also* complication.

skin irritation (due to radiation), 33, 76, 89, 98

sperm, 7, 127, 156, 161

spinal anesthesia, 60

spread (of cancer), *See* metastasis.

staging (of cancer), 16

stress incontinence, 38, 154

stricture, 39, 161. *See also* urethral stricture.

supplement, 5, 19, 32, 104, 109, 114, 117, 138, 141

support group, 22, 26, 33, 48, 122

surgery (prostatectomy), 2, 4, 5, 15, 16, 17, 23, 26, 27, 29, 32, 33, 34, 34, 36–37, 39, 40, 42, 43, 48, 49, 51, 52, 53, 57, 61, 62, 66–67, 71, 72, 74, 79, 81, 84, 90, 91, 96, 102, 103, 107, 110, 111, 112, 113, 116, 117, 118, 120, 122, 125, 126, 127, 129, 130, 132, 134, 135, 137, 139, 141, 148, 151, 152, 153, 154, 155, 156, 157, 161. *See also* laparoscopic prostatectomy; radical prostatectomy, robotic-laparoscopic prostatectomy; salvage surgery; transperineal prostatectomy.

survival rate, 22, 39

Technetium, 8, 10. *See also* radioactive isotope.

technician, 8, 10, 11, 133, 137, 144, 156

template for cryotherapy, 79; for seed placement, 60

tenesmus, 88

testes/testicles, 7, 73; cancer of, 123, 127, 137; removal of (orchiectomy), 73

testosterone, 22, 73, 128, 152, 153, 155

toxicity, 120, 121

transperineal prostatectomy, 151
tumor, 2, 4, 15, 16, 22, 24–25, 27,
  29, 30, 31, 33, 45, 46, 60, 72,
  78, 80, 84, 91, 120, 132, 133,
  145, 149, 159, 160, 161, 162;
  brain, 122; testicular, 123

ultrasound, 18, 22, 56, 58, 62, 70,
  74, 79, 84, 159. See also BAT
  ultrasound machine.
ultrasound probe (for needle
  biopsy), 2, 18, 79
urethra, 26, 39, 48, 61, 66, 67,
  79, 80, 91, 113, 159, 162
urethral irritation, 112, 113, 117,
  119
urethral narrowing. See urethral
  stricture.
urethral sphincter, 63, 67, 69, 86
urethral stricture, 23, 38, 39, 83,
  116
urgency, bowel/rectal, 40, 69,
  70, 81, 82, 87, 89, 92, 97,
  101, 110, 128, 147, 153, 155;
  bladder/urinary, 5, 10, 34, 56,
  61, 69, 70, 81, 82, 87, 88, 89,
  92, 97, 100, 101, 104, 105,
  106, 107, 110, 112, 117, 118,
  119, 122, 124, 128, 134, 161
urinary complications. See complications.
urinary frequency. See frequency.
urinary incontinence. See incontinence.
urinary obstruction, 34, 161

urinary tract infection, 4, 12, 16,
  116, 154
urinary urgency. See urgency.
urination, pain or difficulty
  with, 34, 61, 72, 156
urologist, 1, 3, 5, 15, 18, 21, 26,
  28, 33, 36, 39, 42–43, 48, 66,
  70, 71, 76, 77, 80, 81, 96,
  100, 104, 110, 111, 112, 118,
  119, 122, 125, 127, 132, 135,
  145, 148, 154, 156, 157

vaccine (for treating prostate
  cancer), 121, 122
vacuum pump (for erectile dysfunction), 16, 103, 151
Viagra, 16, 76, 103, 116, 151, 153,
  155
vitamin C, 59, 81
vitamin E, 5, 16, 108–109, 114

watchful waiting, 16, 32, 84, 148

Zoladex, 73. See also hormonal
  treatment.